FREDERICK WALKER MOTT

HISTOLOGICAL OBSERVATIONS

ON

SLEEPING SICKNESS AND OTHER TRYPANOSOME INFECTIONS

Elibron Classics
www.elibron.com

Elibron Classics series.

ISBN 0-543-96961-4 (paperback)
ISBN 0-543-96960-6 (hardcover)

This Elibron Classics Replica Edition is an unabridged facsimile of the edition published in 1906 by John Bale, Sons & Danielsson, Ltd., London.

REPORTS OF SLEEPING SICKNESS COMMISSION.—No. VII.

HISTOLOGICAL OBSERVATIONS

ON

SLEEPING SICKNESS AND OTHER TRYPANOSOME INFECTIONS

BY

F. W. MOTT, M.D., F.R.S.

(*From the Pathological Laboratory of the London County Asylums*)

London

JOHN BALE, SONS & DANIELSSON, LTD.

OXFORD HOUSE

83-91, GREAT TITCHFIELD STREET, OXFORD STREET, W.

DECEMBER, 1906

15.

Histological Observations on Sleeping Sickness and other Trypanosome Infections.

By F. W. MOTT, M.D., F.R.S.

(From the Pathological Laboratory of the London County Asylums.)

(Plates I—XI.)

It is now generally accepted that Sleeping Sickness is a chronic disease caused by the *Trypanosoma Gambiense*, the usual mode of infection being by a biting fly, the *Glossina palpalis*.

Material Used.

By the desire of the Committee of the Royal Society on Tropical Diseases, Colonel Bruce gave instructions to his assistants, and they have forwarded to me from Entebbe material from :—

(1) Twenty-four cases of sleeping sickness in natives.

(2) Portions of the brains of eight monkeys experimentally inoculated with *T. Gambiense*.

(3) Two oxen infected with Jinga trypanosome (probably a species of Nagana), and one donkey infected with mule trypanosome.

(4) The tissues of a monkey that died two years after infection by *T. Gambiense*, which showed the typical lesions of sleeping sickness recorded by Captain Harvey and Major Leishman.

(5) The brain of a rabbit that died three months after inoculation with Surra.

(6) The tissues of two European cases of sleeping sickness. The results of one case under the care of Sir Patrick Manson have been recorded. The histological examination of the other case, for the material of which I am indebted to Dr. Rose Bradford, will be published in full later, although it may be remarked that the results entirely confirm previous observations.

The tissues have been preserved in Formol or Formol-Müller solution, or they have been sent already embedded in paraffin after having been hardened for a short time in 5 per cent. formalin solution. Sections were cut of either 5 or 10 μ thickness.

STAINING METHODS.

The following staining reagents were used for the sections cut in paraffin :

(1) Romanowsky, Leishman, Polychrome blue and eosin. These stains were relied on to show the existence of trypanosomes or their degenerated products, lymphocytes, plasma cells and other cells in the meningeal and perivascular infiltrations. It was found that the polychrome blue and eosin also revealed the glia cells because the body of the cell and processes stain pink, the nucleus blue. These staining methods served also in conjunction with the Gram method for the discovery of micro-organisms.

(2) Heidenhain hæmotoxylin, Van Giesson and modified Mallory and Weigert methods were used for differentiating the neuroglia cells and their processes.

(3) The Marchi and New Weigert methods for showing the acute and chronic nerve fibre destruction. For this purpose the material was embedded in celloidin.

By one or several of these methods combined, observations were made regarding the following points :

(*a*) The existence of trypanosomes, degenerated products of trypanosomes or Leishman bodies.

(*b*) Changes in the nerve cells of the brain, spinal cord and spinal gangli.

(*c*) Changes in the pia-arachnoid membranes, the blood vessels and lymphatic structures especially with reference to (1) the endothelial cells, (2) the neuroglia cells, the branches of some of which form the supporting trabeculæ of the perivascular lymph spaces, and (3) the lymphocyte and plasma cell infiltration characteristic of sleeping sickness.

(*d*) The existence of micro-organisms.

(*e*) The degeneration of nerve fibres and glia substitution.

It may be mentioned that in a number of instances sections of the lymphatic glands, some of which were removed during life and others *post-mortem*, were examined by the same method. The principal pathological conditions observed were either drawn or photographed.

An epitome of most of the cases is given in the form of an Appendix to this communication, together with reference to notes and observations made at Entebbe by the members of the Commission under whose care the cases were. Also observations and notes made by myself on the examination of the tissues.

PART I.

INTRODUCTION.

IN every case of sleeping sickness in which symptoms of the disease were observed during life, I have found the same chronic meningo-encephalitis which I first described in 1898, and which has been since confirmed by the Portuguese Commission, and others. I did not in those two cases find evidence to support the view that this disease was caused by microbial infection, but in the material received since from Uganda, I was surprised at the large proportion of cases, nearly 80 per cent., which showed diplo-coccal or diplo-streptococcal infection. It is therefore not to be wondered at that the Portuguese authorities should at first have considered this organism the essential cause, or that Castellani should, before he discovered the trypanosoma in the cerebro-spinal fluid, have considered the diplo-streptococcus a specific micro-organism for this disease; or that he should have regarded it afterwards as playing an important part in producing secondary or terminal infection and causing the death of the patient, —with which I was myself in agreement. But numbers of facts have accumulated, conclusively establishing the etiology of the disease, (1) the death of Europeans suffering with *T. Gambiense* infection long after they have left the country where the disease is endemic; (2) the production of the characteristic lesions in monkeys by experimental inoculation; (3) the absence of the lesion in any other conditions of infection than trypanosome infection; (4) the chronicity of the disease as shown by European cases; (5) the existence of cases of sleeping sickness only when the *T. Gambiense* and the *G. palpalis* co-exist, as first demonstrated by Colonel Bruce. There is therefore no doubt that the trypanosome infection is *alone* the cause of the disease; but how the trypanosomes produce this characteristic, we might say specific, morbid change in the central nervous system we do not know. Nor has either histological examination or experiment so far solved the question.

There is a parallelism between the intensity of the lethargy, the chronicity of the disease, and the characteristic histological changes in the central nervous system.

Personal observations during life on cases which died in England, and reference to the symptoms and their duration, of cases at Uganda, convince me that the above statement is true, for I have found by microscopical examination of the tissues that those cases which showed the most pronounced cell infiltration of the membranes and the perivascular spaces were the most chronic, and exhibited during life most severe lethargy, *vide* cases 619 and 21. Whereas one case, which had long suffered with *T. Gambiense* in the blood and enlarged glands, but which manifested no signs of lethargy (viz., Bara Risgallah, p. 31), died after a ten days' illness from pneumonia and pneumococcic meningitis, the brain and cord showing no perivascular cell infiltration in those situations where, in sleeping sickness, it is most abundant, namely, the subcortical white matter and the internal capsule.

The tissues of Dr. Bradford's case of sleeping sickness in a European who had left Africa five years, and had therefore certainly suffered with trypanosome infection for that period of time, showed much more chronic and extensive histological change than the nervous tissues of Sir Patrick Manson's patient, who died of sleeping sickness in less than three years after leaving Africa. My observations, however, serve to show that secondary microbial invasion of the blood was the immediate cause of death in the latter case not long after she had commenced to manifest signs of sleeping sickness (*vide* Bibliography).

Morbid Changes in Lymphatic Structures.

The disease is characterised by a chronic polyadenitis (Greig), which is subsequently followed by a chronic inflammatory change in the lymphatics of the brain and spinal cord.

All the observers from the earliest time have noticed the enlargement of the lymphatic glands; and Greig, at my suggestion, punctured the glands and examined the fresh juice. He is of opinion, from his observations, that this is an easier and more reliable mode of determining the existence of *T. Gambiense* than examination of the blood or cerebro-spinal fluid. Dutton and Todd came to the same conclusion working in the Congo State. Many natives in Uganda and the Congo State have, however, enlarged glands, and yet are not the subjects of sleeping sickness. They may be, however, and probably in nearly all cases are, candidates for the disease.

ERRATA.

In referring to the two European cases on pp. 6 and 10 there is an error. Dr. Bradford's case survived exactly three years after leaving Africa. Sir Patrick Manson's case died just under two years after leaving Africa.

Do the trypanosomes get into the glands and *multiply there*, setting up a chronic inflammatory process which terminates in fibrosis? The glands may be inflamed and enlarged, and yet be sterile as regards micro-organisms. It is probable that the trypanosomes infect the lymphatic glands by escaping from ruptured capillaries, or they may become infected by the cerebro-spinal fluid when this secretion contains trypanosomes. Similarly by capillary hæmorrhage the trypanosomes may infect the cerebro-spinal fluid and the lymphatic structures of the central nervous system. If the trypanosomes can set up chronic inflammatory changes in the lymphatic glands, (as there is no doubt they do), and microscopic examination of sections reveals but occasional and scanty evidence of their presence, it is quite reasonable to suppose that they can similarly produce chronic inflammatory changes in the lymphatic structures of the central nervous system. We do not know if the trypanosomes produce this chronic irritation by their mere mechanical presence, which seems unlikely, seeing that the vessels may be crammed with trypanosomes in Nagana and Surra, without causing lymphangitis. There is, according to Plimmer, Thomas and Anton Breine, however, no experimental evidence that trypanosomes produce a chemical toxin; although that would seem the most probable cause of the chronic inflammatory change. The numbers of trypanosomes found in the cerebro-spinal fluid are in no way proportional to the changes found in the central nervous system. Yet there is considerable evidence (*vide* Sleeping Sickness Reports, Royal Society), to show that not until trypanosomes are found in the cerebro-spinal fluid does the chronic inflammatory change take place. If they existed in abundance instead of sparsely, we might consider that this fluid afforded a suitable medium for their propagation, and the absence normally of leucocytes in this fluid might be accounted a cause. On the other hand, the small quantity of proteids which the cerebro-spinal fluid contains would not admit of suitable nutrition.

The posterior spinal ganglia always show some chronic changes, proliferation of the endothelium of the lymphatic capsules of the ganglion cells, together with interstitial lymphocyte accumulation; and these chronic changes may be due to the absorption of toxins from the neighbouring infected paravertebral glands.

In practically all cases of sleeping sickness, the cervical glands are enlarged, and the most chronic change is found about the base of the brain. Hence a probability that the chronic inflammation of the lymphatics spreads along the nerves, spinal ganglia and roots to the central nervous system, and especially along the lymphatics of the nerves and vessels entering the base of the skull. Examination of other tissues, *e.g.*, the heart, pericardium, liver, alimentary canal and testicles, shows, though, generally speaking, in far less degree, an infiltration and accumulation of lymphocytes in the lymphatics, suggesting a defensive reaction. In fact, it might be considered that there is for a long period of time a struggle between the phagocytes and the trypanosomes in the blood, and it is not until the former commence to succumb in the defensive struggle of the organism, that the symptoms of sleeping sickness become pronounced. Certainly in very chronic cases I have been struck by the few polynuclears to be seen in the transected blood vessels as compared with small and[1] large-celled mononuclears, even when the patient has died with terminal microbial invasion.

The chronic inflammatory change of the nervous system is manifested by a proliferation and overgrowth of the neuroglia cells, especially of those which are related to the subarachnoid space and perivascular lymph spaces, with accumulation and probably proliferation of lymphocytes in the mesh work. In chronic cases plasma cells of Marscholko, similar to those in the lymphatic glands, may be found. Various other cells are met with in less numbers, some being the result of degenerative changes and others of endothelial origin, and possessing a phagocytic activity. The characteristic morbid change affects the soft membranes and the vessels.

The membranes.—By the several differential staining methods employed, sections of the cerebral cortex, the base of the brain, the cerebellum and the spinal cord exhibit a chronic leptomeningitis. The chronic inflammatory process is most marked where the cerebro-spinal fluid is most abundant, and it consists of cell proliferation and cell infiltration.

The neuroglia.—There is a marked subpial felting in the molecular layer of the cortex in chronic cases; and in all cases there is some degree of subpial and septal proliferation of the neuroglia. It is not merely an increase numerically of the neuroglia cells, but an increase in size of the body of the cell, and increase in the number and thickness of the processes. In chronic cases it may be almost

---

[1] These large-celled mononuclears are the result of proliferative activity in the red marrow of bone. This tissue was not sent to me, but I have had the opportunity of examining bone marrow from one or two cases.

as pronounced as in some cases of general paralysis (*vide* figs., Plates II and III, and figs. 3 and 5, Plate IX).

Cell infiltration.—The irritative process affecting the arachnoid serous membrane is manifested not only by proliferation of the neuroglia cells contained in the adjacent nervous substance, but also by a proliferation of the endothelial cell-nuclei and an infiltration of the pia arachnoid membrane with lymphocytes which may become transformed into plasma cells of Marscholko. All stages of transition from a lymphocyte to a plasma cell can be seen just as in the inflamed lymphatic glands (*vide* fig. 4, Plate IV, and fig. 2, Plate I). These plasma cells, which are found more often in the perivascular infiltrations, have a characteristic appearance and staining reaction. As the cytoplasm of the lymphocyte grows the nucleus with its wheel-like chromatin particles remain at one end of the cell, and a clear halo separates one side of the nucleus from the cytoplasm. The nucleus stains blue, the cytoplasm pink (*vide* fig. 4, Plate IV).

The vessels.—The striking feature of this disease, distinguishing it from all other chronic nervous affections with which I am familiar, is the universal perivascular cell-infiltration of the central nervous system (*vide* fig. 3, Plate II). This infiltration is most marked and appears earliest in regions where the cerebro-spinal fluid is most abundant. It is therefore very marked about the vessels of the medulla and pons, the cerebellum and the arteries which perforate the base of the brain. It exists around the vessels of the whole of the pia corticalis and spinalis and is obviously related to the lymphatic system (*vide* plates and photomicrographs). As a rule I think the infiltration is more pronounced in the deep sub-cortical white matter than elsewhere. This may be due to the fact that the vessels of the deep sub-cortical white matter have a different source and distribution, and their surrounding lymphatics drain into the subarachnoid space at the base of the brain. An examination of any vessel in a well advanced case reveals characteristic appearances (*vide* figs., Plates I, II, and III). The infiltration under a high power is seen to consist of an extensive proliferation and increase in size of the neuroglia cells, which by their branching processes form the sustentacular framework (*vide* figs., Plate I, and figs. 1, 2, 3, 4, Plate II). Entangled in the mesh work are the lymphocytes and proliferated nuclei of the glia cells or endothelial nuclei.

The relative proportion of lymphocytes to the neuroglial and endothelial nuclei varies in different cases. There are other cells, viz., plasma cells of Marscholko (*vide* fig. 3, Plate I), also large round or oval cells with the nucleus staining deep blue and pushed up to one end or pole, the cytoplasm consisting of a number of clear spherules stained by eosin, giving the cell a mulberry appearance; hence I have called these cells morular cells. They correspond to the Körnchenzellen of Alzheimer. The appearance of these cells suggests degenerated plasma cells. Similar cells are seen in the degenerated structures of infected lymphatic glands. Besides these granulation cells, the result of degenerative processes, there are large macrophages containing red blood corpuscles in various stages of dissolution (*vide* fig. 5, Plate III). These macrophages containing blood corpuscles, when found in the subarachnoid space, indicate hæmorrhage into the cerebrospinal fluid, and suggest that this is the mode in which this fluid becomes infected by the trypanosomes.

Some degree of perivascular neuroglia proliferation was found in two cases of experimental sleeping sickness, when there was no obvious lymphocyte infiltration around the vessels. I have observed neuroglia proliferation in all cases of human sleeping sickness. The more chronic the case the more marked, as a rule, is the neuroglia proliferation; moreover, not only are the neuroglia cells more numerous but they are larger, and with more branching processes (*vide* fig. 1, Plate II). In the monkey, which showed the typical lymphangitis of the central nervous system characteristic of human sleeping sickness, the neuroglia proliferation was more marked than the lymphocyte infiltration. I have had the opportunity of examining the tissues of two European cases; one, which survived five years after leaving Africa, in which sleeping sickness symptoms were observed for more than twelve months; and the other, Mrs. S., who only survived three years after leaving Africa, and in whom sleeping sickness symptoms only existed a few months, death being brought about by diplococcal infection. Comparative observations showed that the former case exhibited much more advanced morbid changes in the lymphatics of the nervous system.

Whence come the lymphocytes in the perivascular spaces? We know that in chronic cases both the small and large mononuclears increase in the blood and the polymorphonuclears diminish; indeed, in some of the very chronic cases transections of the vessels showed hardly any polymorphonuclears, even though there had been a terminal diplo-streptococcal infection. Sometimes quite a number of small and large mononuclears can be seen amidst the red blood corpuscles of transected vessels (*vide* fig. 1, Plate I). There is a considerable difference of opinion whether lymphocytes can migrate by diapedesis; according to Schultze and Ehrlich they are incapable of exhibiting amœboid movements. Ranvier, however, has observed amœboid movements in the lymphocytes squeezed from lymphatic glands, and Jolly has observed amœboid movements in lymphocytes taken from the thoracic duct.

It is very difficult to assert that the lymphocytes seen in the blood of vessels in sections do pass through the walls of the vessels. Certainly the appearances suggest that this may be the source of the lymphocytes in the cerebro-spinal fluid in sleeping sickness and other chronic diseases of the nervous system. There is, however, no proof that they do. What other hypothesis can be offered for this vast accumulation of lymphocytes in the perivascular lymph channels and spaces? The arachnoid space may be considered to be a serous sac, and there is a very close similarity in the appearances presented by the perivascular lymphatics of the nervous system in sleeping sickness, and the perilymphangeal nodules of developing lymphoid nodules of the omentum described by Klein, and figured in Quain's "Anatomy." The serous membranes and lymphatic channels and clefts of other organs may be affected in this disease, as shown by accumulations of lymphocytes (*vide* figs. 2 and 3, Plate X).

The meningeal and perivascular cell proliferation and infiltration of the central nervous system may be regarded as the result of a chronic irritative process connected with the presence of the trypanosomes in the cerebro-spinal fluid.

This cell proliferation and infiltration is made up of proliferated branching neuroglia cells, in which are entangled lymphocytes and proliferated endothelial nuclei and possibly young neuroglia cells with a small amount of cytoplasm. The origin of the lymphocyte infiltration is uncertain; it may be (1) that the lymphocytes come from the blood by diapedesis or by rupture of vessels, and having entered the cerebro-spinal fluid proliferation takes place; (2) that they accumulate in the obstructed lymph channels of the perivascular lymphatics; they may be formed by the proliferating nuclei of the lymphatic endothelial cells, the same as they appear to be in lymphatic glands. But besides, there is the chronic inflammation of the lymphatic glands, generally terminating in fibrosis, which may obstruct the drainage of the cerebro-spinal fluid from the closed cerebro-spinal cavity along the lymphatics of the cranial and spinal nerves. Universal chronic inflammation of the lymphatic glands terminating in an obstructive fibrosis would tend to block the flow of the cerebro-spinal fluid and lead to accumulation of proliferating lymphocytes.

There is considerable difficulty in distinguishing between nuclei of glia cells and lymphocytes. The chromatin particles of the glia cells, usually two or three, lie in a pale nucleoplasm. The nuclei of the neuroglia cells are, as a rule, larger than lymphocytes (*vide* fig. 4, Plate II, and fig. 4, Plate X). They undergo active proliferation not only in the perivascular spaces but in the tissues. The young glia cells lie in pairs, or fours, or more, and may have but little cytoplasm surrounding the nucleus.

Examination of slides of the fresh juice of the glands obtained during life by puncture and stained for trypanosomes, proves conclusively that the cause of the glandular enlargement and of the chronic inflammatory changes met with, is the presence of trypanosomes. Yet the microscopic evidence of the existence of trypanosomes in the sections of the glands is not more satisfactory than the evidence of their existence in the perivascular and meningeal infiltration of the nervous tissue. Chromatin particles which may be micronuclei and macronuclei can be seen as well in one as in the other, and smears of fresh brain sometimes reveal trypanosomes just as the smears of glands.

Smears of glands removed during life from the necks of natives suffering with *T. Gambiense*, but not yet manifesting signs of sleeping sickness, *although sterile as regards micro-organisms*, showed trypanosomes and degenerated products of trypanosomes in the form of small and large chromatin rings (macronuclei and micronuclei). Sections of the same glands exhibited macronuclei and micronuclei and, occasionally, a trypanosome. As the glands were sterile, it may be presumed that the trypanosomes were the cause of the swelling and chronic inflammatory changes. The sections showed increased vascularity and lymphocytes in all stages up to the formation of large plasma cells of Marscholko (as shown in fig. 4, Plate IV.), and large numbers of degenerated swollen plasma cells like those seen occasionally in the perivascular lymph spaces of the brain in sleeping sickness. Moreover, some of the large cells appeared to be endothelial cells which have taken on a phagocytic function and eaten up lymphocytes and chromatin particles. The endothelial cells have proliferated in these inflamed glands, and there is a tendency to fibrosis, nuclear proliferation and thickening of the trabeculæ and walls of the lymph sinuses and vessels. Latér these glands, when the inflammation subsides, become fibrous, dense and less vascular. Quite similar appearances were observed in glands removed during life from the neck in cases of pronounced sleeping sickness. These glands were frequently sterile, but the majority which I received that were removed *post mortem*, and quite a number even removed during life, showed points of suppuration in their interior, and an infection with diplostreptococci. I have, however, come to the conclusion that these organisms only play the part of a terminal or late secondary infection due to the breaking down of the defences of the organism. This diplostreptococcal invasion must, however, play an important part in hastening the fatal termination.

In a discussion which took place at the meeting of the British Medical Association at Toronto, August, 1906, when I demonstrated the histological changes in the nervous system of some chronic trypanosome infections, Professor Welch called attention to the fact that Councilman had shown that in every fatal case of small-pox streptococcal invasion occurred. He asked whether the absorption of microbial toxins could be absolutely excluded as a cause of the histological changes. In reply I stated that, undoubtedly, the fatal termination was hastened in a large number of cases by the microbial invasion, and my observations had shown that a systematic examination of the lymphatic glands had led to the demonstration of organisms where microbial invasion had not been suspected. Yet the etiology of the disease and the study of some of the chronic fatal cases, and particularly the European case under the care of Dr. Bradford, showed that the trypanosomes, apart from microbial invasion, caused the characteristic changes in the nervous system.

In marked chronic cases of sleeping sickness the appearances presented by the lymphatic glands resemble in many ways the infiltration of the perivascular lymphatics of the central nervous system. In the latter there are proliferated lymphocytes, granule cells, plasma cells, proliferating endothelial cells, occasional degenerated trypanosomes and numerous chromatin particles, many of which are probably micronuclei and macronuclei, entangled in the markedly proliferated neuroglial sustentacular framework. Figs. 4 and 5, Plate V., show this correspondence of the histological appearance in the lymph sinus of the gland and the perivascular lymphatics of the brain.

We may therefore conclude that the presence of the trypanosomes in these perivascular lymphatics in the subarachnoid space (as evidenced by their constant existence in the cerebro-spinal fluid, sometimes in such numbers as to be found without centrifuging) might cause, as in the lymphatic glands, this chronic lymphatic inflammation of the central nervous structures. Infection of the cerebro-spinal fluid may be from the lymphatic glands, or more likely from the blood by capillary hæmorrhages. The European cases and the few animals which have shown the characteristic lesions have all lived over eighteen months after infection; it consequently takes time to effect the change. Lymphatic gland-enlargement is characteristic of all forms of chronic trypanosomiasis of animals.

All cases of sleeping sickness have trypanosomes in the cerebro-spinal fluid at some time or other, and it is probable that the entrance of the trypanosomes into this fluid marks the onset of, and slowly causes, the chronic inflammatory change in the lymphatic system of the central nervous system. The alternative hypothesis is that the trypanosomes, by multiplying in the lymphatic glands, produce a toxin which is absorbed by the lymphatics, and this toxin proceeds along the vessels and nerves to the lymphatics of the cerebro-spinal axis, the route being especially from the cervical glands by the lymphatics of the large vessels and nerves entering the base of the skull.

This chronic inflammation of the lymphatics of the brain with perivascular glia cell proliferation, lymphocyte and plasma cell accumulation gradually and progressively interferes with the flow of the lymph stream and the circulation of the cerebro-spinal fluid. It is not decided whether the cerebro-spinal fluid functions as the lymph of the brain, or whether it simply forms a water jacket around the lymphatic sheath which is closely applied to the wall of the blood-vessel. The lymphocytes and glia cells certainly fill up this space and interfere with the normal outflow of the fluid from the cerebro-spinal cavity; consequently when lumbar puncture is performed there is usually evidence of increased pressure; moreover the fluid contains abundance of lymphocytes. This increased intracranial pressure interferes also with the circulation of the blood in the small vessels, and the characteristic symptoms of the disease, viz., lethargy, tremors and muscular weakness, may be explained by the functional depression of the nerve cells from a deficient nutrition and interference with oxidation processes, brought about by mechanical and bio-chemical interferences with the activities of the nerve cells, and not by neural destruction. This is shown by the patients retaining comprehension of their surroundings and by their intelligent response to questions when roused from their lethargy. A totally different picture to general paralysis (also a meningo-encephalitis) in which there is a profound parenchymatous change, whereas sleeping sickness is *a primary interstitial process;* although later on in the disease, especially when it is chronic and of long standing, marked chromolytic cell changes and a certain amount of destructive degeneration of the neurons do occur.

CHANGES IN THE SMALL VESSELS AND CAPILLARIES.

The capillaries in the pia and in the brain tissue show the following changes, but these are not nearly so marked as in general paralysis of the insane.

The nuclei of the endothelial cells may undergo proliferation, and in the neighbourhood of the capillaries and small vessels there are often numerous lymphocytes, plasma cells and glia cells; but I fail to find evidence of sprouting new capillaries as seen in general paralysis, nor can I but very rarely find any evidence of the Stäbchenzellen or rod cells described by Alzheimer, and regarded by him as very characteristic of this disease. These Stäbchenzellen, I consider, are probably collapsed capillaries (*vide* fig. 6, Plate II).

Capillary hæmorrhages are met with in all forms of trypanosome disease, and probably are the result of obstruction by the organisms.

CHANGES IN THE NEURAL ELEMENTS.

Although the meninges are in many cases obviously thickened and the convolutions flattened (indication of some intracranial pressure), yet there is no naked eye wasting of the brain. The depth of the grey matter of the cerebral cortex is not appreciably diminished, although the vessels both in the grey and white matter may appear somewhat congested. In very chronic cases, after the brain has been hardened in formol-Müller solution, then washed in water, the transections of the vessels may appear like dark dots surrounded with a pearly grey ring. The dark centre is due to the blood contained in the vessel, and the surrounding zone of a pearly grey colour is due to the perivascular cell infiltration.

I have not observed granulation of the ependyma of the ventricles, so characteristic of the meningo-encephalitis of general paralysis of the insane. Moreover the wasting of the grey matter of the cerebra cortex, so characteristic of this disease, is not met with in sleeping sickness. The convolutions are broad and of normal size, and the sulci tend to be obliterated in sleeping sickness; whereas in general paralysis the convolutions are shrunken from atrophy of the neural elements, cells and fibres, and the sulci are consequently broad and deep. In both diseases there is obvious meningeal thickening, and septal and perivascular changes, but here it seems to me the similarity ends. But this statement becomes more apparent and convincing when the microscopic changes are described. Moreover, a comparison of the size of the remaining structures of the central nervous system show that in general paralysis there is a primary neuronic atrophy which does not occur in sleeping sickness. Thus to the naked eye the spinal cord in the latter disease may appear normal as regards amount of grey and white matter, whereas in general paralysis the cord is often much reduced in size, and there is very obvious neuronic atrophy.

The naked eye appearances therefore point especially to a primary parenchymatous degeneration in general paralysis with chronic interstitial and meningeal inflammation, whereas in sleeping sickness the morbid change is primarily interstitial and with some secondary parenchymatous atrophy.

Microscopic Examination of the Nerve Cells and Fibres.

Cells.—Stained by the various modifications of Nissl method, sections of the various structures of the central nervous system, viz., cortex cerebri, cerebellum, pons, medulla oblongata and medulla spinalis, also spinal ganglia, exhibited certain changes, but in comparison to the interstitial perivascular and meningeal change they were inconsiderable, thus contrasting markedly with general paralysis.

Let us consider, firstly, the cortex cerebri. Under a low power, the five layers of Meynert can usually be easily differentiated. The most obvious change is in the subpial molecular layer of Cajal, but the three layers of pyramids above the layer of granules are usually distinctly seen, the cells usually retaining their pyramidal form, their apical processes being straight as a rule, and the cells arranged in columns, a picture quite different to that seen in general paralysis.

The abnormal feature, apart from the perivascular infiltration, is the abundance of nuclei of neuroglial cells and lymphocytes scattered about and often lying in groups in the perineuronal spaces (*vide* photomicro).

The great majority of the specimens of nervous tissues from sleeping sickness cases which I have examined, have shown marked changes in the ganglion cells of the central nervous system when examined under a high power. I have reason to believe that these changes are largely due to the effects of secondary or terminal microbial infection, to pyrexia, or in some cases, hyperpyrexia. But a terminal or secondary microbial invasion with toxæmia and fever would produce universal effects, and in such cases one finds that throughout the nervous system the ganglion cells present a chromolytic change, the whole ganglion cell staining with polychrome and eosin a diffuse purple, and showing an absence of the Nissl pattern of the cytoplasm. In the first case I examined in 1898, the patient died of septic hyperpyrexia from an abscess in the lung. Although the interstitial meningeal and perivascular change was most pronounced, the neuronic degeneration was comparatively slight, although the patient was in the third stage of the disease. The outline and shape of the ganglion cells of the central nervous system did not present marked changes, but every cell showed a diffuse chromolytic change. This was obviously due to the high fever. Nevertheless, in chronic cases marked chromolytic changes and atrophy of dendrons do occur in the ganglion cells, especially in those regions where the perivascular infiltration is most severe, and where, in consequence, a certain amount of blood stasis takes place. I have observed this in the medulla oblongata; and the affection of the important cardiac and respiratory centres in this region may, in a few uncomplicated cases, be the ultimate cause of death. The changes in the ganglion cells may therefore be considered as due (1) to the primary lymphangitis, and (2) to secondary microbial toxæmia. It is difficult to differentiate the cells which are affected by the one cause from the other.

I consider, however, that the chronic change is indicated in those cells in which (1) there are appearances of atrophy of the dendrons, the protoplasmic processes being either attenuated or broken off; (2) the cytoplasm still exhibits some remnants of a pattern of Nissl granules in the circumference of the cell and on the dendrons; (3) the nucleus is large and clear and often eccentric. Sometimes a dead ganglion cell may be seen being devoured by phagocytes (*vide* figs., Plate VI). The cells of the spinal cord usually show much less change than the cells of the medulla oblongata and cerebral cortex. The cells of the posterior spinal ganglion usually show chromatolysis, but not destruction (*vide* fig. 1, Plate VII).

The appearance of the cells in acutely fatal trypanosome infections, *e.g.*, Surra and Jinga in animals, could be accounted for by the anæmia caused by the blood change and the obstruction of the small vessels by the trypanosomes. In the brain of the rabbit dying of Surra, the ganglion cells all showed a shrinking of the cytoplasm, a marked chromatolysis and disappearance of the Nissl granules, and swelling of the nucleus, and a change not unlike that observed in some forms of experimental anæmia (*vide* fig. 3, Plate VIII).

Changes in the Central Canal of the Spinal Cord.

Not only is there evidence of a chronic irritative action of the cerebro-spinal fluid by the cell proliferation in the meningeal and perivascular lymphatics, but in all chronic cases the central canal of the spinal cord is filled up owing to a proliferation of the cells of the ependyma. I found this had occurred in quite juvenile subjects. It was so in the little Congo negro boy, who died in Charing Cross Hospital in 1898, and I was of opinion then that this fact afforded evidence of a very chronic nervous affection caused by some irritating agent (*vide* fig. 1, Plate X). It was the same with the juvenile cases from Uganda, Sempagana, aged 8, Hamesi, aged 12, and Kaperi, aged 8-10. Such change denotes, then, a chronic process of considerable duration. It is probable in the light of our present knowledge of the possible long duration of the disease that these subjects were infected when quite infants.

Examined under a high power, the nuclei of the cells lining the spinal canal may often be seen undergoing active proliferation, and specimens stained with polychrome and eosin exhibit large pale nuclei with a thin membrane and chromatin granules stained blue surrounded by a pale pink amorphous substance. In the grey matter around the central canal numerous glia cells having a similar appearance can be seen.

Examination of the Central Nervous System for Fibres by Weigert and Marchi Methods.

In cases uncomplicated by terminal microbial infection there is a certain amount of fibre atrophy proportional to the cell atrophy described. This atrophy is most obvious in the tangential layer of the cortex cerebri, where the fibres in places are greatly diminished, or even absent. There may also be some diminution of the fibres in the super-radial and inter-radial systems, especially in chronic cases. There is, however, in the brain as in the spinal cord, no definite system-tract sclerosis, the result of atrophy of a neuronic system (*vide* figs. 1, 2, 4, Plate IX). Generally in the lateral columns corresponding to the pyramidal systems some degenerated fibres can be seen by Marchi method, but the glia proliferation tends to follow the distribution of the septa rather than to accord with any definite atrophy of a system of nerve fibres (*vide* fig. 5, Plate IX).

By Marchi method, the cerebrum, cerebellum, spinal cord and spinal ganglia were examined in a number of cases. In most instances the results were unsatisfactory owing to a generally diffuse blackening of the myelin sheaths and the deposition of black granules. I consider this change[1] was probably the result of acute changes in the myelin, brought about by terminal microbial toxæmia, fever, &c. Some few of the cases, however, did not show this generalised change in the myelin, and a certain number of fibres showing Wallerian degeneration were found. These changes we may regard as definite and indicative of neuronic decay.

The results above described tend to show that a chronic trypanosome infection of the cerebro-spinal fluid causes a meningo-encephalitis and myelitis characterised by a chronic interstitial inflammation of the lymphatic structures of the central nervous system, and the cell proliferation induced thereby precedes and is far in excess of the parenchymatous change, contrasting markedly therefore with the meningo encephalitis of general paralysis. It resembles general paralysis by the infiltration around the vessels of lymphocytes and plasma cells and by the neuroglia proliferation.

In sleeping sickness, even in advanced stages of the lethargy, the patient when aroused comprehends and responds in an intelligent manner to questions, proving that his associative memory is intact. Although he readily becomes fatigued and his speech and movements are tremulous, denoting impairment of highest motor innervation, yet there is no evidence of dementia as seen in general paralysis.

These clinical facts, which broadly separate these two diseases, entirely accord with the pathological changes. The neural elements in sleeping sickness are functionally impaired by the interstitial change, but when the patient is roused the neural elements of mind are still capable of functioning for a short time in a normal manner. But in general paralysis, where the interstitial change is less marked but the parenchymatous degeneration is progressive and destructive of neural elements, the mind is proportionally incapable of functioning normally.

---

[1] I have observed this in other diseases when there has been an infective process, especially when the tissues have been placed in formol-Müller. I do not, therefore, attach much importance to it.

In conclusion, it may be asked, If the trypanosomes are the cause of this chronic inflammation of the central nervous system, why are they not found in the infiltration and in the blood in sections?

The *T. Gambiense* is only found by careful search in blood films. They are seen with great difficulty in sections unless they exist in the blood in considerable numbers.

Secondary or Terminal Microbial Invasion.

After death, in the great majority of the cases which I have examined secondary or terminal microbial infection had occurred.

Sometimes the diplococci were found in sections of the blood vessels as well as in the membranes, indicating a generalised infection (*vide* fig. 2, Plate V., and fig. 6, Plate IV).

The culture experiments of Novy and McNeal show that infection of the culture media by micro-organisms interferes with the growth of the trypanosomes. The cases in which I found trypanosomes in the blood contained in sections of vessels of the nervous system, were two chronic cases uncomplicated as far as I know by microbial infection. In the European case, under the care of Sir Patrick Manson, the histological investigation of which Low and I reported, the trypanosomes disappeared from the blood a short time before death; this was coincident with a generalised diplo-streptococcal invasion.

How far diplo-streptococcal invasion of lymphatic glands may generate toxins without general blood infection and induce chronic changes in the lymphatics of the central nervous system I am not prepared to say.

The fact that swollen glands in the neck removed during life are sterile does not prove that other glands in the body, which cannot be removed are sterile. Deep seated glands may be infected by micro-organisms. Possibly it may be shown that as long as the body is able to resist bacterial invasion the trypanosomes are unable, by themselves, to produce the changes which cause sleeping sickness. There is, however, vere little evidence of this hypothesis, and it must be assumed that in some way (which we have not at present discovered) the trypanosomes, or some modified form of them, set up this lymphangitis of the central nervous system. When there was an invasion of the central nervous system by diplococci, it seemed probable that this occurred by way of the lymphatics proceeding from infected paravertebral glands. Sections of the cervical nerves, spinal ganglia and posterior roots in some cases enabled me to trace the course of the microbial infection (*vide* fig. 1, Plate IV).

PART II.

Experimental Evidence.—Animals inoculated with *T. Gambiense* usually die before the characteristic lesions of the nervous system can occur. I have examined the tissues of nine animals (monkeys) which were inoculated at Entebbe in one way or another with *T. Gambiense.* They were all said to have exhibited the characteristic lethargy, but it is very difficult to differentiate (according to my experience) between a monkey that sits moping when profoundly ill, and an animal which exhibits a lethargy on account of the brain lesion.

The tissues of the brains of all the animals sent to me, with the exception of two, showed no characteristic change. The vessels of the brain were empty and there was no meningeal or perivascular infiltration. Several of these animals had survived the infection (as proved by the existence of trypanosomes in the blood) one year. One was subsequently infected with diplo-streptococcus from a sleeping sickness case; yet there was no sign of the meningo-encephalitis met with in every case of human sleeping sickness. This was the experience apparently of Ayres Kopke.

(1) The tissues of one monkey inoculated with *T. Gambiense* showed, however, the characteristic lesion of human sleeping sickness. This case was reported by Major Leishman and Captain Harvey. It survived the infection eighteen months. I have examined portions of the tissues kindly given to me by Major Leishman and find that there is a very marked neuroglia proliferation of the perivascular lymphatics, endothelial cell proliferation and lymphocyte accumulation, and a few plasma cells around the vessels of the brain in all the situations examined. In fact, the lesion in no respect differs essentially from that of human sleeping sickness (*vide* fig. 2, Plate III). The cerebro-spinal fluid and tissues in this case were, according to Leishman, sterile.

(2) A monkey, upon which large numbers of infected flies were allowed to feed on several successive occasions, exhibited trypano-

somes in the blood and cerebro-spinal fluid, and died eight months after the first fly feeding, having presented symptoms of lethargy. Reports of the Sleeping Sickness Commission of the Royal Society, No. VI., pp. 107 and 108.

The subcortical white matter of this animal showed a considerable glia cell proliferation in relation to the vessels (*vide* fig. 1, Plate III), but there was little evidence of lymphocyte accumulation. The spinal cord also showed a glia proliferation (*vide* fig. 3, Plate IX). It is possible, therefore, that the glia cell proliferation precedes the lymphocyte accumulation in the perivascular spaces.

(3) Monkey 99. The medulla oblongata and tissues about the base of the brain showed a commencing subpial, septal and perivascular glia proliferation.

Examination of the nervous tissues of animals inoculated with Nagana, Surra and Jinga trypanosomes, and which died within a few months of infection, the blood swarming with trypanosomes, or modified or degenerated trypanosomes, showed no perivascular or meningeal changes.

(1) The brain of a rabbit inoculated with Surra, which died three months later, was kindly given me by Dr. Plimmer, and showed the following appearances in sections. By any of the staining methods employed nearly all the blood-vessels showed masses of trypanosomes, as the coloured drawings exhibit (*vide* figs. 2, 3, and 4, Plate VIII). Single trypanosomes could be seen in the capillaries; in the larger vessels solitary trypanosomes and whorls of trypanosomes and plasmodial masses, which are either degenerated trypanosomes consisting of a zoogl\u0153al mass in which many deeply-stained macro-nuclei and micro-nuclei can be seen, or of am\u0153boid forms, described by Plimmer and Bradford. But in spite of this extraordinary trypanosome infection the blood-vessels showed little or no inflammatory reaction. The perivascular lymph spaces showed no lymphocytes; and the ganglion cells showed only marked chromolytic changes; otherwise there was nothing noteworthy in the nervous system.

(2) The brains of two oxen infected with Jinga trypanosomes were examined. The animals died within three months of infection; the results of the examinations were extremely interesting and will be given in some detail.

Experiment 162 (*loc. cit.*, p. 171).—The cortex cerebri, the cerebellum, medulla and spinal cord were examined, and all yielded the same results. With a magnification of 1,200 diameters, the capillaries and vessels were found to contain chromatin bodies closely resembling Leishman bodies, except that they were smaller, measuring from 1 to 2 μ, much more frequently 1 μ, rarely as large as 2 μ. They were either circular or oval rings, or had the appearance of the chromatin particles situated at the two poles. Several drawings from photomicrographs are given to illustrate their appearance and their numbers. Some of the capillaries show immense numbers, and in some transections of larger vessels these bodies may be observed lying in a zooglœal mass (*vide* figs. 3, 4, and 5, Plate VII).

Individual bodies exhibit some diversity in their form, indicating division. A large number of stained particles (which may be micro-nuclei) can be seen.

The Jinga trypanosome, as the accompanying drawing shows (*vide* fig. 2, Plate VII), is comparatively a large organism, as seen in the blood of a monkey, which was inoculated with it. Its oval macro-nucleus is much larger than these chromatin bodies which are seen in the vessels. If these chromatin bodies, as Leishman would affirm, are the macro-nuclei of trypanosomes, then it is difficult to explain why a dozen or more of the chromatin bodies can sometimes be seen lying in a space which could be covered by one trypanosome. Still, the trypanosomes may have degenerated elsewhere and the macro-nuclei have been carried into the capillaries. In view, however, of the researches of Captain Rogers regarding Leishman bodies being altered phases of trypanosomes, and the contention of Plimmer and Bradford *re* the existence of amœboid forms of trypanosomes, it is possible that these chromatin bodies may be some phases in the life of the trypanosomes in the blood. For comparison a drawing is given of the appearances presented by Leishman bodies in the spleen and splenic blood from preparations kindly lent by Sir Patrick Manson. The preparations were made from a fatal case of Kala-Azar.

Experiment 202 Ox (*loc. cit.* p. 174).—This animal died within three months of infection. Portions of the brain were stained in bulk by polychrome and eosin and sections cut 5 μ thickness after embedding in paraffin.

In this way the contents of the vessels were but little disturbed so that trypanosomes existing in the serous fluid contained in the blood vessels were recognisable in great numbers. The appearances of the trypanosomes and their modified forms are seen in fig. 1, Plate VIII.

It may be mentioned that in these two cases there was no sign of meningo-encephalitis, and there was no diplo-streptococcal infection. The ganglion cells showed chromolytic changes, and there were *many minute capillary hæmorrhages*, probably due to plugging of the capillaries by the organisms. I have frequently observed in the lymphatic glands, meninges and perivascular lymphatics of the brain of sleeping sickness, chromatin rings, very similar to, only smaller than the chromatin rings seen in the vessels of Jinga and Surra infected animals, of the trypanosomic origin of which there can be no shadow of doubt. It is therefore probable that a number of the chromatin particles seen in the tissues of sleeping sickness are all not *débris* of degenerated cells but *débris* of degenerated trypanosomes or their modifications. Especially would this argument be valid if the tissue, as in the case of the glands removed during life, had been shown to be sterile. Moreover, I have seen appearances in sections of lymphatic glands removed during life, of threadlike attenuated forms of trypanosomes resulting from division, not unlike those figured by Gray and Tulloch as multiplying by fission in the stomach of the *G. palpalis* (*vide* figs. 1 and 2, Plate V).

The experiments on animals, together with the examination of the central nervous system of a horse that died of dourine more than two and a half years after infection (a full account of which has been published in the **Proceedings of the Royal Society*, B., Vol. 78, 1906), tend to show that chronic trypanosomiasis is attended by a chronic lymphatic irritation. This irritation is manifested in the nervous system by a neuroglia proliferation, and subsequent lymphatic proliferation and accumulation.

Animals that die within a few months of inoculation have not survived a period of time long enough to manifest this neuroglia proliferation.

It is probable that animals infected directly by blood from sleeping sickness cases containing *T. Gambiense* might, if they were inoculated in the abdomen or hind legs, show changes in the spinal cord before they showed changes in the brain. This may account for the fact that Plimmer's rats only showed changes in the spinal cord; and in dourine or *mal de coit* the changes in the central nervous system are

* Since the above was published Dr. Lingard has kindly forwarded to me from the Imperial Bacteriological Laboratory of India the nervous tissues of other animals that have died of Dourine, wherein I have found the same change, though less marked.

primarily and most markedly severe in the lumbo-sacral region of the spinal cord, especially of the posterior and lateral columns.

Further experiments on animals should, in my opinion, be carried out, anthropoid apes being used, and the neck should be chosen as the seat of inoculation.

In conclusion, I have to thank my assistant, Mr. Chas. Geary, for valuable assistance in making the microscopic preparations, and Miss Agnes Kelley for assistance in making preparations, especially for the very accurate and beautiful drawings illustrating this Report.

I have appended a short report of the changes in the glia tissue of sleeping sickness by Dr. Georg Eisath (see next page).

ADDENDUM.

A Detailed Description of the Neuroglia Changes in the Brain and Spinal Cord of Eight Cases of Sleeping Sickness. By Dr. Georg Eisath, Hall, Tyrol.

Dr. Eisath has for some time past been investigating the changes in the neuroglia by a special differential method of staining, which he has described in a communication entitled "Ueber normale un pathologische Histologie der Menschlichen Neuroglia." *Monatsschrift für Psychiatrie und Neurologie.* Band xx.

As he was working upon this subject in my laboratory, I placed at his disposal the nervous tissues of eight cases of human sleeping sickness which, by reason of their condition and mode of hardening and preservation, were suitable for staining by his method.

Subjoined is a translation of the account which he has kindly sent me of the results he obtained. They confirm and amplify the observations which I have described in this Report.

To Dr. Eisath is due the credit, by his differential method of staining, of showing the relative importance of the glia cell proliferation in the perivascular infiltrations and the quantitative relationship of glia nuclei to lymphocytes in this disease.

(1) *The character of the glia cells and their differentiation from lymphocytes.*—(*a*) The nuclei of the glia cells almost universally show a distinct nuclear membrane and possess normally two to three nuclear bodies, besides other small granules. The leucocyte nuclei are of many forms; some are round and possess an abundance of granules, others are lobulated and have an indistinct outline.

(*b*) The glia nucleus forms quite one-third of the transverse diameter of the cell, whilst the nucleus of the leucocyte fills up the greatest part of the cell. That is to say, the glia cell has a relatively much larger proportion of cell protoplasm than the leucocyte.

(*c*) The protoplasm of the glia cell is arranged in a star-like manner around the nucleus; and the border of the cell, in normal conditions, is very distinctly seen, whilst in the leucocytes it is not.

(2) *The distribution and localisation of the glia proliferation.*—The glia overgrowth is demonstrable in every case and the cells are

both increased in numbers and size. Giant glia cells were observed, and in every case the Weigert fibres are increased.

In the molecular layer of the cortex of many cases the glia cells are increased and often show an abundant formation of Weigert fibres, especially around the vessels. In the Meynert ganglion cell layers the increase of glia cells is relatively much less developed than in the superficial layer of the cortex, and in the white substance. The Weigert fibres, moreover, are only sparingly seen. In one case (Kirongo) the fibre formation is hardly demonstrable, and glia cells with surrounding protoplasm and processes are hardly recognisable in the cortex. The glia overgrowth in the white substance is, however specially observable around the larger vessels. *It exists not only around those vessels which show leucocytic infiltration, but also around capillaries where infiltration with round cells has not occurred.*

In the medulla oblongata the overgrowth and the morbid changes are most extensive.

In the spinal cord an extensive overgrowth of glia tissue exists by which the individual nerve fibres are surrounded, and this overgrowth affects all the tracts as well as the grey matter. There is no appreciable outfall of the medullated fibres, *only here and there and quite sparsely have the medullated fibres disappeared.* The glia cells are numerically increased and increased in size beyond the normal.

(3) *Pathological changes in the glia cells.*—The glia granular substance was not precisely investigated in this work and shows, so far as the researches extend, in the round glia cells *no marked pathological changes.*

Isolated glia cells possess well developed protoplasmic processes, others enormously increased Weigert fibres. Some of the glia cells have a uniform *homogeneous stained protoplasm* as if the nuclear substance had dissolved out or had disappeared.

Such cells usually have a dark brown stained nucleus, whilst others may have lost their processes and are converted into *hyaline balls.*

APPENDIX.

Notes of the Cases of Sleeping Sickness and Animals Experimentally Inoculated, with the Principal Facts Observed on Microscopic Examination of the Tissues.

(*a*) Brief abstract of notes of clinical records.
(*b*) Microscopical examination of tissues.
(*c*) Remarks.

1. Nabujam, aged 30; died April 4, 1903. Sent as a case of sleeping sickness, turned out to be a case of tumour cerebri. No trypanosomes.

Microscopical Examination. — No meningo-encephalitis; no micro-organisms.

2. Zakibu. Admitted March 22, 1903.—Enlarged glands, tottering gait, temperature normal, no tremors. April 14.—General convulsions, left facial palsy. April 16.—Death. Trypanosomes in cerebro-spinal fluid; pneumonia—pneumococcal invasion of blood. Brain surface injected; Subarachnoid fluid excess—dull and opaque; no sign of active or acute meningitis. The substance of the brain appears healthy to the naked eye.

Microscopical Examination. — Chronic meningo-encephalitis; pneumococcic invasion; vessels of brain in places plugged with cocci.

3. Nonbi. Admitted February 23, 1903.—States that three brothers and four sisters all died of sleeping sickness. April 18.—General condition: Enlarged glands, no *trophic changes*. She is well nourished; pronounced nervous symptoms. She is conscious and tries to answer questions, but cannot. She lies all day absolutely torpid, with her eyes open. There is slight lateral nystagmus—pupils equal, no reaction to light; twitching of muscles, knee jerk absent, no ankle clonus. Died April 20.—Trypanosomes in cerebro-spinal fluid. *Post mortem.*—No signs of pneumonia; pericarditis. Brain: Dura mater normal; convolutions of the surface of the brain are flattened, the sulci filled with opaque-looking subarachnoid fluid; the vessels are injected, otherwise nothing abnormal.

This is an ordinary case of sleeping sickness. The anæmia may have been helped by ankylostomata. The pericarditis is an uncommon feature; meningo-encephalitis, peri-vascular infiltration very marked; great numbers of diplococci in the membranes—between the cells and in the leucocytes; well-marked advanced glia proliferation, especially of deeper layers of cortex and subjacent white matter. Microscopic examination indicates a chronic case.

4. Kaperi, aged 8 to 10 years.—Trypanosomes in the cerebro-spinal fluid. Case of purulent meningitis. Remarks: "In our experience these acute inflammatory cases are not usual. In this case it is evidently due to streptococcal invasion. This appearance is not typical of sleeping sickness: as a rule, there are no signs of acute inflammation, but merely a flattening of the convolutions, an injection of vessels, and an excess of subarachnoid fluid" (p. 39, vol. i., Sleeping Sickness Reports).

Brain and spinal cord: No glands or other tissues sent; acute diplo-streptococcic meningitis, the whole of the meninges affected; mostly a polymorpho-nuclear exudation; not much extension to perivascular lymphatics of the nervous substance in the cortex and spinal cord, but fairly well marked in the medulla oblongata and base of brain (probably the primary seat of the infection by the micro-organisms). In the medulla oblongata there are vessels in which the inflammatory exudation shows numbers of mononuclear leucocytes, and amorphous red-stained granules of varying size from 1μ to 2μ or more—probably the result of coagulation necrosis of the broken-up chromatin particles of the polymorpho-nuclear leucocytes, and also the diplococci in their capsules. No trypanosomes seen in any of these sections. The ganglion cells show acute chromolytic and coagulative necrotic changes.

5. *Dr. Nabarro's Case.*—Some material was sent to me by Dr. Nabarro. The patient died of pneumonia. The ordinary meningo-encephalitis, characteristic of sleeping sickness, was found, and diplococci in the blood of transected vessels and in the inflammatory products.

6. Dreya. Case 69, E. E.—Admitted February 6, 1903; died June 12, 1903. A chronic case (*vide* fig. 1, Plate XI). Trypanosomes were obtained by lumbar puncture on June 2. Appearances of brain typical of sleeping sickness. Central nervous system examined: no lymphatic glands sent. All the appearances of a chronic meningo-encephalitis. Very marked perivascular infiltration of the whole central nervous system, especially of the base of the brain and medulla oblongata. No polymorpho-nuclears seen in the inflammatory exudation, which consists almost entirely of proliferated glia cells of mononuclears and plasma cells of Marscholko, also a number of morular cells. The exudation, as seen in the drawing, is most extensive, and extends to the smallest vessels, leading to their obliteration in some instances. The capillaries are seen often to contain yellow amorphous material instead of corpuscles. In the meningeal infiltration, also in the perivascular lymphatics are seen a great number of granule bodies of various sizes. It was thought that some of these granules might be the products of degenerated trypanosomes, as appearances like a macro-nucleus and micro-nucleus occasionally were seen. The great majority of the granules were, however, probably products of coagulation necrosis of nuclear chromatin particles of dead cells. The ganglion cells, especially of the medulla oblongata, were profoundly changed. The dendrites were broken off, the perikaryon pale, and either devoid of Nissl granules or were broken up; the nucleus was swollen, clear, pale, and often eccentric. The pigment was increased; all these changes pointed to a chronic degenerative change, which *may be* due to the action of the noxious agent which produces the inflammatory change, but more likely the result of nutritional defects occasioned by the vascular changes. Very occasionally a transected vessel would show a portion of a trypanosome, and one vessel showed, in addition, a whole organism.

7. *Case* 248.—Suleman Bin Mahomed, aged about 45 years, Persian, the first Asiatic to be affected at Entebbe. Came originally from Bushire on Persian Gulf. October 28.—History: Has been in Africa twenty years, of which he spent the first two years in East Africa. Has been in Uganda, on and off, for eighteen years, and has been down to the coast twice in that time. Latterly he has been a "headman" in the Government Transport Department, and when at Entebbe has lived near the lake. In fact, for some time he has lived almost like the natives and with them. He became ill two months ago, and was then seen by Dr. Hodges, whose report is as follows:—

September 2.—There are general tremors, anæmia, slight pyrexia (temperature 100° F.). Weak, irregular, rapid pulse. Spleen slightly enlarged. Left otitis media. Blood films examined, malaria found. October 28.—Lumbar puncture performed. Numerous trypanosomes seen in first field. Many lymphocytes. No red blood corpuscles.

October 31.—Present state. Patient is a very tall man, obviously wasted and ill. There is a heavy, sad look about the face and eyes, *vide* photograph. General condition very weak and feeble; gait weak and staggering. Voice weak. Marked tremor of tongue and lips. Slight tremor of fingers and hands. There is a fairly marked tremor of the body and head. No enlarged glands about neck, slight in groin (due to sore feet). Has pain in left ear, due to otitis media. Pulse fair tension, 68 per minute. Knee-jerks sluggish. Heart sounds feeble, no bruit.

November 6.—Photograph taken (*vide* fig. 2, Plate XI). November 12.—Patient has improved to a certain extent since he has been in hospital. Died later.

The brain showed the typical characters of sleeping sickness. No glands sent.

Microscopical Examination.—Chronic meningo-encephalitis fairly advanced. Not much change in form of the ganglion cells of the cortex; Meynert's columns fairly well seen, but obvious acute toxic change, as all the cells stain diffusely with the blue and erythrosin a dull purple—doubtless, an acute toxic change due to terminal microbial infection. Many of the transected vessels show plugs of streptococci—I have never seen so many in the blood in any condition previously; short bacilli are seen also in great abundance in the perivascular spaces (*vide* fig. 6, Plate III).

In the remaining cases the deep paravertebral glands of the neck, and often other lymphatic glands, were forwarded at my request, together with the adjacent nerves and posterior roots and ganglia, from a good few of the cases.

8. Case 69, Q. Q.—This was described as an acute case of sleeping sickness. No other notes.

Lymphatic glands: Paravertebral cervical glands filled with diplo-streptococci, and in places causing points of suppuration. Great plugs can be seen in the lymph channels, and no doubt the escape of these into the blood stream led to the general infection and death. Other parts of the gland show signs of chronic inflammation and necrosis; plasma cells are abundant, also granules of varying size. No definite trypanosomes seen. Posterior spinal ganglion with commencement of cerebro-spinal nerve and spinal roots from cervical enlargement near the glands above described. There is a very marked perivascular infiltration; the capsules of the cells are also crammed with lymphocytes and the small vessels hardly observable normally in the roots and the mixed cerebro-spinal nerves are now readily discernible by the abundance of mono-nuclear cells accumulated in their lymphatic sheaths. The loose vascular connective tissue around the ganglion is also crowded with lymphocytes. Diplococci and streptococci with capsules are seen everywhere along the course of the lymphatics; in some places they form a regular injection (*vide* fig. 1, Plate IV).

Central nervous system: There is a generalised meningo-encephalitis throughout, more marked in the cerebellum and around the perforating vessels of the basal ganglia and internal capsule than elsewhere. Many small vessels are seen plugged with organisms (*vide* fig. 2, Plate IV), and there are, in consequence, numerous small foci of softening. In these foci, which are microscopic, are found ganglion cells which have undergone coagulation necrosis, lymphocytes and broken-down cell *débris* and granules. Everywhere in the cells and between the cells of the inflammatory products there are diplococci and streptococci. There are no plasma cells seen. The nerve cells show generally acute changes, some are stained dull purplish throughout, exhibit no Nissl bodies, have crumbling edges, and their dendrons destroyed. Some of the nerve cells exhibit the appearances associated with a more chronic toxic condition, viz., the perikaryon is stained diffuse pink and exhibits no Nissl bodies, whereas the outer part of the cell is stained blue from remaining Nissl bodies; the nucleus is generally pale, swollen and eccentric; the borders of the cells are curved outwards instead of incurved, and the processes are either broken off or diffusely stained.

Remarks.—I do not possess notes of this case, for beyond the statement that it was acute, no information was sent. It appears to me, however, that the acute course of the disease was due to the streptococcal invasion, firstly of the glands and secondly of the cerebro-spinal fluid and blood. The former may have been infected by the lymphatics of the nerves, and this doubtless gave rise to the acute symptoms; but, probably from the appearance of the ganglion cells and the abundant glia proliferation and perivascular mono-nuclear infiltration, there was a source of chronic irritation, non-microbial in origin. The glands show chronic changes also.

9. Bara Risgallah (male), aged 35 years; occupation, police. Lives in hut in police lines. A case which for some time had been under observation with trypanosome fever and enlarged glands. The notes state that trypanosomes were readily found in the gland juice, and they were actively motile. The stained smears show, in addition to the fully-formed tryanosomes, structures which were evidently altered trypanosomes. I am informed that acute symptoms developed and the patient died of pneumonia after ten days' illness. It was stated in the *post mortem* notes that possibly a pneumococcic meningitis would be found. The glands *post mortem* were found to contain diplo-streptococci, but not those removed *intra vitam*. Captain Greig informs me that the cerebro-spinal fluid in this case had shown mono-nuclear leucocytes.

Microscopic Examination. — A number of smear preparations of the glands were sent, and trypanosomes found. *Glands* removed *intra vitam* showed the following characters (*vide* figs. 3 and 4, Plate IV.).

(1) Numbers of granules, probably *débris* of cells and their nuclei, uniformly stained a dull pink; occasionally bodies which might be considered *débris* of trypanosomes and their macro-and micro-nuclei were found, and one trypanosome entire was seen (*vide* fig. 2, Plate V).

(2) Lymphocytes in all stages of transition to the plasma cells of Marscholko can be seen. Lastly, degenerative changes of the plasma cells.

(3) Proliferated and degenerated endothelial cells.

(4) Spaces filled with deep blue stained coagulated lymph. Glands removed *post mortem* showed the same appearances, but diplococci were present.

Cerebrum, Cerebellum, Medulla Oblongata and Spinal Cord. — The meninges, especially of the cortex and base of brain and the cerebellum, were the seat of an acute pneumococcic meningitis. There was little or no perivascular infiltration with mono-nuclears; the cell exudation consisted almost entirely of polynuclears. There was no obvious glia proliferation, as seen in the other cases. Cervical spinal ganglion and nerve: Lymph spaces and lymphatics packed with cocci in great abundance. Smear preparation of spleen: No trypanosomes, granules, or micro-organisms found. Smear preparation of the centrifuged cerebro-spinal fluid: No trypanosomes; diplococci, small and large mono-nuclears, and a few red corpuscles. Smear preparation of brain: No trypanosomes found, abundance of diplococci.

Remarks.—The clinical history of this case coincides with the facts obtained by histological investigation. A chronic inflammation of the lymphatic glands associated with trypanosome infection, secondary diplococcal infection of the glands, pneumonia and pneumococcic meningitis, possibly occasioned by the defences of the organism against invasion having been destroyed by the chronic glandular affection. The absence of any obvious signs of chronic irritation of the central nervous system in the form of glia proliferation and perivascular lymphatic mononuclear infiltration may be correlated with the absence during life of any definite degree of sleeping sickness.

10. Tabula (male), aged 25. Entebbe. Occupation, marine. A chronic case of Trypanosoma Gambiense infection with enlarged glands, but not yet affected with signs of sleeping sickness. The lymphatic glands removed *intra vitam* exhibited inflammatory changes with necrotic foci similar to the glands of Bara Risgallah.

11. 69, L. L., and **12,** 69, K. K. In both of these cases there was suppuration in the deep suboccipital and cervical glands found *post mortem*, which in some cases had broken down, forming cavities. This was especially marked in the glands near the cranium (along the vessels), and those near the spinal cord. Pure cultures of diplo-streptococci were obtained from both of these cases from the cerebro-spinal fluid and heart blood.

Microscopical Examination of Brain Spinal Ganglia and Roots.—No micro-organisms were found in the brain, but abundance of diplo-streptococci in the lymph spaces of the posterior roots and spinal ganglia, also in the blood vessels of the sheath of the ganglion, and in the lymph spaces of the nerves of neck. The perivascular mononuclear infiltration is fairly evident in the central nervous system; amidst the cells are numbers of granules of varying sizes.

13. 69. J. J. Axillary, femoral and glands of receptaculum chyli. Chronic and acute inflammatory changes, necrotic areas, diplo- and diplo-streptococci, also *Filaria perstans* in abundance.

14. 69, G. T., Masake. Admitted May 6, 1904, died May 24, 1904. Aged 16. Active trypanosomes in cervical glands. Blood also showed trypanosomes in films. No streptococci. *Post mortem* cultures from glands of neck. No streptococci.

Microscopical Examination of Tissues.—Intense chronic perivascular infiltration and glia proliferation about cerebellum and medulla (*vide* figs. 2, 3 and 4, Plate I), less obvious of cortex, very marked in cervical posterior spinal ganglia, nerves and roots. Large numbers of granules which take capsular stain. Lymphatic gland adjacent: To the naked eye (after hardening in Müller-formalin fluid), there appears to be yellow necrotic areas. Sections stained by Gram show crowds of small foci of diplo-streptococci, also in a polychrome section a transection of a vessel shows diplo-streptococci surrounded with polynuclears.

15. 69, R. R., Abimerika (male), aged 22. Admitted February 27, 1904, died June 11, 1904. The gland juice was examined on June 4, and showed active trypanosomes. No diplococci cultivated in broth and agar. *Post mortem:* No diplococci in glands. Heart's blood showed pure culture of *Bacillus coli communis.*

Microscopical Examination.—All sections of glands sent showed abundance of diplo-streptococci. Cortex, cerebellum and spinal cord show advanced chronic meningo-encephalitis, abundance of granules and occasional definite diplococci at the base of the brain; especially about the cerebellum there are foci of streptococci in the chronic inflammatory products, as if a reinfection had occurred. Transections of the blood vessels in the medulla oblongata showed a very intense perivascular infiltration, consisting of proliferated glia cells, lymphocytes, and many plasma cells and morular cells with granular *débris.* A trypanosome was seen in a transected vessel in this case. The ganglion cells have undergone profound chronic degenerative changes. This was a chronic case, and the microscopic appearances were quite in conformity, for there was marked cell degeneration and glia proliferation.

16. Sempagama (male), No. 237. Aged 8. Admitted October 10, 1903; died June 15, 1904. A very chronic case. Trypanosomes very abundant in glands, blood and cerebro-spinal fluid during life. "*Post mortem:* There was a large clot of blood over left hemisphere of brain between the dura mater and brain surface. No hæmorrhages internally. Day of death total leucocytes 74·680, polynuclears 42, and small mononuclears 43. Red blood corpuscles, 3,000,000, Hb. 70 per cent."

Microscopical Examination of Tissues.—Chronic meningo-encephalitis of brain and cord. Well marked diplo-streptococcal infection of meninges of base of brain and of the perivascular infiltration. Numerous granules, many of which take capsular stain; they lie in a sort of pink stained amorphous substance, and it was thought that gradations between diplococci in their clear capsules to organisms which had undergone death and become merged into their capsules could be seen.

17. Case 69, K. P., Arcadi (male), aged 25. Admitted May 17, 1904: died July 27, 1904. Many trypanosomes in glands. Diplococci were obtained from glands about ten days before death. Deep cervical glands show points of suppuration.

Microscopical Examination.—Glands showed acute and chronic inflammatory changes in all the glands examined. In all the glands that were suppurating were abundant streptococci and necrotic areas, but in the glands that were not suppurating were numerous foci of diplococci. No definite trypanosomes could be seen in the sections, although frequently a body looking like macronucleus and micronucleus was seen. Pieces of *Filaria perstans* were also seen.

Chronic Meningo-encephalitis — plasma cells — glia proliferation and degeneration of the ganglion cells. Amidst the degeneration products are bodies which may be degenerated trypanosomes, also bodies which are probably dead and swollen up diplococci, and here and there can be found distinct diplococci.

18. 69, F. V., Hamesi (male), aged 12. Admitted May 5, 1904; died July 24, 1904. A rather acute case. There was a terminal streptococcal invasion, many trypanosomes in glands and blood.

Microscopical Examination.—Chronic meningo-encephalitis. Proliferation of nuclei of capillaries. Perivascular infiltration of lymphocytes, plasma cells and morular cells, with marked glia proliferation. No trypanosomes. Streptococci in the vessels and in the membranes of the pia corticalis. One lymphatic gland sent. No organisms found, but several nodules of the gland show acute inflammatory changes with many polymorpho-nuclears and coagulated fibrin.

19. 69, V. V., Wasiwa (male), aged 18. Admitted January 1, 1904; died July 22, 1904. A very chronic case. Pure trypanosome infection. No streptococcal invasion.

Microscopical Examination.—Gland taken post mortem contains abundance of streptococci not in blood vessels. Gland taken *intra vitam*, apparently plugs of cocci not numerous. Brain shows chronic meningo-encephalitis fairly advanced. A marked glia proliferation.

20. Dumani, male, aged 20. Admitted April 25, 1904; died May 19, 1904. Trypanosomes found in cervical glands, April 25, 1904. No streptococci.

Post mortem.—Streptococci not detected, but broken down trypanosomes in gland.

Microscopical Examination. — Glands. Plugs of diplo-streptococci in sheath of gland and especially around vessels of hilum. The gland itself does not show much change. Apparently this gland has been infected secondarily to another gland in the chain which was not sent. Degenerated trypanosomes (?). Chronic perivascular meningo-encephalitis. Miliary hæmorrhages in spinal cord. Morular cells which apparently in some instances appear to be endothelial macrophages filled with altered corpuscles (*vide* fig. 5, Plate III).

21. Case 69, Z.K., Msubika (female), aged 7. Admitted June 10, 1904, died August 12, 1904. On admission patient was in an advanced stage of the disease; she had a terminal diplo-streptococci infection. Glands were generally enlarged and in left submaxillary region showed points of suppuration.

Microscopical Examination.—Very chronic advanced meningo-encephalitis (*vide* figs. 1, 2, and 3, Plate II). To the naked eye, after hardening in formol-Müller solution the brain does not show a change like general paralysis. The cortex is of good depth, but the vessels are easily discernible, both in the grey and white matter, especially in the latter are they visible, by points and streaks of semi-translucent, grey, gelatinous appearance, with often a dark central core of blood.

The microscopic examination showed an intense meningeal and perivascular infiltration of proliferated branching glia cells, lymphocytes, plasma cells and morular cells. The cervical glands examined showed chronic inflammatory changes and although there is no suppuration in the glands examined there are abundant foci of diplo-streptococci.

Experiment 56.—Monkey (*Cercopithecus Sp.*), (*vide* p. 33. Report IV. Sleeping Sickness Commission). "To note the effect of the injection into the vertebral canal of blood containing trypanosomes from Case 66, Tabula, Marine." April 14, 1903.—Examined blood of monkey, found malarial parasites but no trypanosomes. Injected by lumbar puncture into spinal canal 2 cc. of blood from Tabula containing trypanosomes. May 7.—Trypanosomes found in the blood of the animal. July 10.—The animal died, having shown no very marked symptoms of sleeping sickness. No temperature chart kept. The *post-mortem* examination was negative. The cerebro-spinal fluid contained living trypanosomes. "Death occurred seventy one days after inoculation, and in our opinion is probably due to the trypanosomes."

Microscopical Examination.—Cerebellum, cortex cerebri and medulla oblongata. No sign of meningo-encephalitis. Very marked acute chromolytic changes in the cells of the medulla, with disintegration. Some change in cells of cortex cerebri but much less pronounced. Slight change in cells of Purkinje. Nearly all the sections show malarial parasites, also diplococci and streptococci; probably a late terminal infection, as there is no evident inflammatory reaction.

Experiment 60.—Monkey (*Macacus rhesus*). "To note the effect of the subcutaneous injection of blood from a case of trypanosome fever." April 15.—Injected subcutaneously 2 cc. of blood containing trypanosomes from Case 66, Tabula, Marine. May 7.—Trypanosomes appeared in the blood for the first time, twenty-two days after injection. May 14.—Noted as being very numerous. July 2.—Up to the present this monkey has shown no signs of being ill. To-day, however, he appears listless and less energetic. July 15—Died. For the last fortnight the animal has presented the same picture of sleeping sickness as noted in the case of Experiment 1, monkey. Picture of the animal with its head sunk on chest. (This attitude is, however, that assumed by all monkeys when ill.—F. W. M.)

Remarks.—Page 33 Sleeping Sickness, Report IV. As far as one could judge this animal presented the typical appearances of sleeping sickness during life, and the brain after death looks like the normal sleeping sickness brain in miniature. The organs showed no disease, so that one is bound to look upon the injected trypanosomes as the cause of death. But the trypanosomes which were injected subcutaneously into this monkey were taken from the blood of a case of trypanosome fever, Tabula, Case 66, who up to the present has shown no signs of sleeping sickness.

Microscopical Examination.—No meningo-encephalitis. A few diplococci seen by Gram's method in the brain. Nothing noteworthy in cerebrum and cerebellum except some chromatolysis of cells. It seems that the large psychomotor cells are especially deficient in Nissl granules. There is some recent glia proliferation, as shown by a comparison of the motor cortex of this animal with that of a Macacus that died from other causes than sleeping sickness.

Experiment 34.—"To note the effect of injecting the cerebrospinal fluid from a case of sleeping sickness into the vertebral canal of a monkey." April 8, 1903.—Injected 1 cc. of cerebrospinal fluid containing trypanosomes from a case of sleeping sickness into the spinal canal of this monkey (male, pale faced variety). April 30.—Trypanosomes appeared in blood.

Remarks.—Four months after inoculation this monkey began to show symptoms of sleeping sickness. Captain Greig writes on September 10 that the animal had died.

Post-mortem was pretty typical of an ordinary sleeping sickness case. Trypanosomes were found living in the cerebrospinal fluid of the brain.

Microscopical Examination.—No meningo-encephalitis. No perivascular infiltration. Blood vessels of brain empty. Endothelial proliferation of capillaries. Marked chromatolysis of cells of cord and medulla, to a less degree of cortex. Glia proliferation.

Experiment 8.—Monkey (*Cercopithecus Sp.*). "To note the effect of injection of blood from trypanosome fever into a monkey, and secondly, the injection of a pure culture of streptococcus from a case of sleeping sickness. The injection of blood was performed twice in April, and repeated in May, 1903. No symptoms of sleeping sickness followed; the following March (nearly a year later) subcutaneous injection of streptococcus culture. No change occurred." August 22, 1904.—It was noticed that the animal is now crouched up, and presents a dull drowsy expression. (It may be remarked that the description of the animal in no way differs from the description of the typical sleeping sickness cases.—F. W. M.) August 28.—The animal died. Trypanosomes were present in the cerebrospinal fluid, *but the fluid was sterile as regards micro-organisms.* Cysts were discovered in the liver and peritoneum, but their nature is not described.

This animal lived nearly eighteen months, apparently the *subcutaneous* injection of the streptococcus had no effect. In the remarks it states that towards the end the animal showed the characteristic signs of the disease. It is assumed that the streptococcus had nothing to do with death.

Microscopical Examination.—The cerebral cortex, medulla, internal capsule, spinal cord and cerebellum were examined. There is no perivascular infiltration or meningitis of the nervous system. There are marked chromolytic changes of the ganglion cells and some acute glia proliferation.

Experiment 99. Monkey (*Cercopithecus Sp.*)—"To observe the effect of infection of the monkey by tsetse flies which had fed on a sleeping sickness patient twenty-four hours previously, and the effect of subcutaneous injection of a pure culture of diplo-streptococcus on the course of this infection."

The feeding was begun on May 15, 1903.

July 23, 1903.—Trypanosomes were noted in the blood for the first time.

January 15, 1904.—Animal out of condition generally, but is still fairly active.

February 14, 1904.—Animal is weak and thin. He is crouched up, and frequently his attitude is very characteristic, the head drooping between his knees.

February 22.—Animal lies about a good deal. He takes his food better. His temperature is still swinging.

March 2.—Subcutaneous injection of pure culture of diplo-streptococcus.

March 19.—Animal is in a moribund condition. Gland in right groin distinctly enlarged; this was removed and found to contain pus. Smears showed, under the microscope, diplococci and "bodies" stained blue, which appeared to be degenerated trypanosomes.

March 20.—Animal died in the night. *Post mortem* 9 a.m. The body is markedly emaciated. Lymphatic glands in both femoral regions are enlarged. Glands in right femoral region are suppurating. Glands in axilla and neck are enlarged but not suppurating. Pupils equal and normal. No increase of fluid in pleural or peritoneal cavities, slight increase in pericardial.

Brain.—On removing the calvarium the dura mater is seen to be normal; on reflecting it, the convolutions are seen to be slightly flattened and the superficial vessels are injected; the subarachnoid fluid is increased, no active trypanosomes were seen microscopically, but the animal had been dead for some time. A pure culture of a streptococcus was obtained from the cerebro-spinal fluid.

Heart.—Nothing noteworthy. Blood from this organ examined microscopically showed many trypanosomes. Malaria is also present.

Lungs.—Both healthy.

Liver, Spleen and Kidneys.—Show nothing noteworthy.

Intestines.—Healthy.

Lymph Glands.—In omentum and mesentery distinctly enlarged.

Remarks.—This experiment demonstrates several points of importance, the first being that it is possible to convey the trypanosma of sleeping sickness from man to monkey after an interval of twenty-four hours; secondly, that the disease produced in the monkey by the fly infection presents the same characters as that produced by inoculation of cerebro-spinal fluid or blood from a case of sleeping sickness. This animal presented towards the close of its life a typical picture of a sleeping sickness case.

The experiment is, finally, of interest and importance from the fact that fifteen days before its death it had been injected with a pure culture of diplococci obtained from a case of sleeping sickness. So far as we could observe, the course of the disease was uninfluenced by the injection, the only noteworthy feature being a slight suppuration in one of the groups of lymphatic glands near the seat of inoculation. Portions of the nervous system and glands have been preserved for minute investigation and the results of the examination will be of interest. (Sleeping Sickness, Report VI., p. 39.)

Microscopical Examination.—In the medulla, cord and brain there was no trace of perivascular infiltration or meningitis found. There was a little chronic inflammatory thickening at one spot of the floor of the 4th ventricle. The marked chromolytic and acute destructive changes found in the spinal cord and medulla of an uneven nature was very striking and resembled the changes seen in Surra rabbit (p. 22) and Jinga trypanosomiasis of ox. In the cord and medulla oblongata also a few capillary hæmorrhages were seen, but a careful search showed no flagellated organisms in the blood contained in the vessels of the central nervous system. Appearances, however, were presented closely similar to those met with in Jinga trypanosomiasis, viz., the capillaries both in transverse and longitudinal section showed oval and round protoplasmic bodies stained pink, measuring from 4 to 10 μ, which contained minute chromatin particles in varying numbers and sizes. In many instances these bodies could be seen lying in the lumen of vessels transversely and longitudinally, also free in the brain tissue. The chromatin particles frequently had the appearance of rings measuring 1 μ and other small particles were frequently seen in the pink stained protoplasm. Those lying in the wall of the vessel or outside it might be proliferated and swollen endothelial or glia cells. Examination of a blood film did not show these bodies although a few trypanosomes were found. There is pronounced glia cell proliferation in the cortex cerebri, especially in the subjacent white matter; also in the cerebellum. The cells are probably young for they have as a rule, few and not extensive branching processes and the cell protoplasm is proportionally scanty.

Experiment 228, p. 106. Reports, Vol. VI. of Sleeping Sickness Commission. Monkey (*Cercopithecus Sp.*).

"To note the effect of the trypanosome carried by tsetse flies freshly caught in the vicinity of Entebbe on a monkey."

The experiment was started on October 12 and a large number of flies fed on the animal, but it we not until November 26 that trypanosomes were found in the blood. Later this no more flies were fed on the animal and it lived until June 19 when it was in a moribund condition and was killed by chloroform. The brain presented no noteworthy naked eye change. The superficial lymphatic glands, both femoral and axillary were enlarged; abdominal slightly enlarged.

Remarks.—This experiment illustrates the course of the disease produced by the trypanosomes carried by the tsetse flies (*Glossina palpalis*) freshly caught in the vicinity of Entebbe. It closely resembles the experiment in which the *Trypanosome Gambiense* was injected into the monkey. In both the course of the disease was a *prolonged* one; the animal in this experiment also showed definite signs for some time before death. At times it presented the characteristic features met with in the sleeping sickness monkeys. The temperature curve was also very similar. This experiment supports the view that the trypanosome carried by the freshly caught tsetse fly in Uganda is identical with the *T. Gambiense*.

Microscopical Examination.—Portions of the brain and medulla were examined. There was no obvious perivascular cell infiltration, but there was a very marked chromolytic change of the ganglion cells of the medulla, somewhat similar to that seen in the Surra rabbit's brain. A considerable degree of acute glia proliferation, especially marked in the subjacent cortical white matter, also in the medulla oblongata (*vide* fig. 1, Plate III).

There is a perivascular glia proliferation especially about the smaller vessels. These cells are larger than normal, star-like, and show many branching processes extending on to the vessels. A portion of the cervical enlargement of the spinal cord with anterior and posterior roots attached, also posterior spinal ganglion and three quarters of an inch of the cerebro-spinal nerve beyond the ganglion with adherent tissue was embedded in paraffin and cut in one block. The sections were stained by the various methods described and microscopical examination proved of considerable interest. The adherent connective tissue attached to and forming part of the sheath of the cerebro-spinal nerve shows a chronic inflammatory change similar in many respects to that observed in the lymphatic glands and perivascular lymphatics of the central nervous system in human sleeping sickness. There is a marked proliferation of the endothelial cells with nuclear proliferation and endogenous nuclear changes, degeneration and necrosis of the cytoplasm of the cells and lymphocyte accumulation. Stained by Gram method no micro-organisms were seen. Stained for trypanosomes, the appearances were exactly like those observed in the lymphatic glands removed during life (and in which active living trypanosomes were found in the juice), viz., occasional appearances which may be due to modified or degenerated trypanosomes. Since this chronic inflammation does not appear to have been caused by microbial invasion and as undoubtedly this animal was infected by the flies with trypanosomes we may conclude that this chronic inflammation of the adjacent structures and sheath of the nerve was due to the trypanosomes (fig. 3, Plate IX).

If the nerve be traced from this inflammatory perineural tissue to the ganglion, small accumulations of lymphocytes can be observed in the lymph spaces, and there is an early interstitial nucleus roliferation in the spinal ganglion, but this is only obvious in scattered pieces. Along the posterior roots there are small scattered accumulations of lymphocytes, but on reaching the spinal cord there is some evidence of chronic irritation by the sub-pial and septal proliferation of the neuroglia tissue. This is most obvious at the ring where the posterior root fibres enter the posterior horn; it extends on the lateral surface, nearly halfway to the anterior median fissure and posteriorly to the posterior median fissure. There is slight proliferation but not so marked in the remainder of the periphery of the spinal cord (*vide* photomicrograph). This distribution suggests that the noxious agent is carried especially by the lymphatics of the posterior roots. There appears to be a commencing glia proliferation of the grey matter generally, but this is not so obvious.

The neuroglia change in this cord closely corresponds with that observed by me in the lumbo sacral region of a horse that died of Dourine (*Trypanosoma equiperdum*).

These observations tend to show that the lymphangitis may extend from the lymphatic glands of the neck along the perineural lymphatics, but prior to this a noxious irritative agent may be absorbed by the neural lymphatics and bring about a neuroglia proliferation. There appears to be an excess of lymphocytes in the grey matter, and here and there accumulations of lymphocytes around the small vessels can be seen. Unless all the lymphatic glands of the body can be proved to be free from microbial infection—consequently absorption of microbial toxins by the neural lymphatics put out of court as a cause of this chronic glia irritation and proliferation—it may always be considered as not proved beyond all shadow of doubt that the trypanosome infection *per se* is the cause.

BIBLIOGRAPHY.

[1] MOTT. "The Changes in the Central Nervous System of Two Cases of Negro Lethargy, sequel to Dr. Manson's Clinical Report," *Brit. Med. Journal*, vol, vi. p. 1666, 1899.

[2] MOTT. "A Case of Negro Lethargy, by Stephen Mackenzie, with a Note on the histological Changes of the Nervous System by F. W. Mott," *Trans. Path. Soc. Lond.*, vol. li., part ii., 1900.

[3] MANSON and MOTT. "African Lethargy, or the Sleeping Sickness," *Trans. Path. Soc. Lond.*, vol. li., part ii., 1900.

[4] MOTT and LOW. "The Examination of the Tissues of a Case of Sleeping Sickness in a European," *Brit. Med. Journal*, April, 1904.

[5] MOTT. "Observations on the Brains of Men and Animals Infected with Various Forms of Trypanosomes," *Proceedings of the Royal Society*, vol. B. 76, 1905.

[6] MOTT. "The Cerebro-spinal Fluid in Relation to Diseases of the Nervous System," *Brit. Med. Journal*, December, 1904.

[7] BETTENCOURT. Kopke, Gomez de Rezende, Correa Mende, "La Maladie du Sommeil," Lisbon, 1903.

[8] WARRINGTON. "A Note on the Condition of the Central Nervous System in a Case of African Lethargy," *Brit. Med. Journal*, vol. ii, p. 929, 1902.

[9] SICARD et MONTIER. "Recherche Bact. et Histol. dans un cas de Maladie du Sommeil chez un blanc," *La Presse Med.*, December, 1905.

[10] CASTELLANI. "Researches on the Etiology of Sleeping Sickness," *Journal of Tropical Medicine*, June, 1903.

[11] BRUCE. "Reports of the Sleeping Sickness Commission."

Vol. I. (1) CASTELLANI. "Presence of Trypanosomes in Sleeping Sickness."

(2) BRUCE and NABARRO. "Progress Report on Sleeping Sickness in Uganda."

Vol. II. (3) CHRISTY. "The Distribution of Sleeping Sickness."

(4) CASTELLANI. "Adult Forms and Developmental Forms of the Trypanosomes found in Sleeping Sickness."

(5) LOW and CASTELLANI. "Report on Sleeping Sickness from its Clinical Aspects."

Vol. III. (6) CHRISTY. "The Epidemiology and Etiology of Sleeping Sickness in Equatorial East Africa."

(7) THEOBALD. "Report on a Collection of Mosquitoes and other Flies from Equatorial East Africa."

Vol. IV. (8) BRUCE, NABARRO and GREIG. "Further Report on Sleeping Sickness in Uganda."

Vol. V. (9) AUSTEN. "A Provisional List of Diptera."

(10) NABARRO and GREIG. "Further Observations on the Trypanosomiases (Human and Animal) in Uganda."

Vol. VI. (11) GREIG and GRAY. "Continuation Report on Sleeping Sickness in Urganda."

(12) GREIG. "Report on Sleeping Sickness in the Nile Valley."

(13) AUSTEN. "The Distribution of Tsetse-flies."

(14) GRAY and TULLOCH. "The Multiplication of the Trypanosoma in the Alimentary Canal of the Glossina Palpalis."

12 THOMAS and ANTON BREINL. "Trypanosomes, Trypanosomiasis and Sleeping Sickness. Report vol. vi., part ii., 1905." Thompson Yates and Johnston Laboratories, University of Liverpool.

13 NOVY. *Journal of Infectious Diseases*, vol. ii., No. 2, March, 1905.

14 KOPKE. "Investigações sobre a Doença do Somno," *Archivos de Hygiene e Pathologia Exoticas*, vol. i., fasc. 1.

15 HARVEY. "Report on a Case of Experimental Sleeping Sickness in a Monkey," *Journal Royal Army Medical Corps*, May, 1905.

16 BRADFORD and PLIMMER. "The Trypanosoma Brucei, the Organism found in Nagana or Tsetse-fly Disease," *Quart. Journal Micro. Science*, vol. xlv., April 20, 1905.

17 ROGERS. "Preliminary Note on the Development of Trypanosoma in Cultures, of the Leishman Donovan Bodies of Cachexial Fever and Kala Azar," *Lancet*, July 23, 1904.

18 MARSHALL. The present state of knowledge is well summed up by Marshall (F. W. M.). "Trypanosomiasis or Sleeping Sickness," *Review of Neurology and Psychiatry*, February, 1906.

19 JOLLY, M. J. "Sur les Mouvements des Lymphocytes," *Soc. de Biol.*, June, 1902.

20 ALZHEIMER. "Histologische Studien zur Differenzialdiagnose der Progressiven Paralyse."

21 PLIMMER. "Note on the Effect produced on Rats by the Trypanosomata of Sleeping Sickness," *Proceedings of the Royal Society*, vol. lxxiv., No. 504, February 24, 1905, pp. 388-390.

DESCRIPTION OF PLATES.

Except where otherwise stated all sections were stained with methylene blue and eosine.

PLATE I.

FIGS. 1-4.—Appearances presented by the vessels of the brain in a very chronic case of sleeping sickness.

FIG. 1.—Transection of small vessel of medulla oblongata, showing perivascular infiltration with hyaline lymphocytes. In the centre of the blood vessel is a trypanosome (*t*). Amidst the blood corpuscles there are numerous small and large mononuclear leucocytes (*mon. l.*). Magnification 500.

FIG. 2.—Small vessel, with plasma cells (*p*) and large granule cells, which I have termed morular cells (*m*). They correspond to Körnchen Zellen of Alzheimer. Magnification 500.

FIG. 3.—Small vessel dividing into two capillaries, showing nuclear proliferation of the endothelial cells; in the neighbourhood are plasma cells (*p*), lymphocytes (*l*), and glia cells (*g*). Magnification 500.

FIG. 4.—Section of spinal ganglion, showing lymphocyte interstitial infiltration (*l*). Magnification 120. Same section is shown more highly magnified in fig. 1, Plate VII.

PLATE II.

FIG. 1.—Three large glia cells (*g*), their branches ending in a network around and upon a small vessel; lymphocytes (*l*), and plasma cells (*p*) are seen scattered about. Magnification 500.

FIG. 2.—Small vessel, showing endothelial nuclei proliferated, and three plasma cells. Magnification 500.

FIG. 3.—A transection of a vessel in a very chronic case of sleeping sickness, showing marked perivascular infiltration. Magnification 250.

FIG. 4.—Active proliferating young glia cells found in great numbers in sleeping sickness tissues. The pale nucleus, with distinct nuclear membrane, contains chromatin granules, with an arrangement indicating mitosis. Surrounding the nucleus is the pink-stained cytoplasm, with a tendency to form star-like processes. Magnification 500.

FIG. 5.—Two large morular cells from a very chronic case of sleeping sickness. Magnification 500.

FIG. 6.—Rod cells (Stäbchen Zellen) are rarely met with, although occasionally appearances like fig. 6 are seen. Magnification 500.

PLATE III.

FIG. 1.—Section of subcortical matter of brain of monkey that died after infection by trypanosomes caused by infected flies being allowed in considerable numbers to bite the animal. Experiment 228. There is little or no perivascular lymphocyte infiltration, but a considerable increase in size and number of the perivascular glia cells. Magnification 430. Stained by Heidenhain method.

FIG. 2.—Section of subcortical white matter of monkey that died eighteen months after infection and which showed the characteristic lesion of sleeping sickness. Harvey and Leishman. The glia proliferation is well seen, and in the meshwork of the branching fibres which form the reticulum of the perivascular lymphatic space (which is seen in longitudinal section) are numerous lymphocytes. The body and reticulum of the glia cells are stained pink in the section; the lymphocytes and neuroglial nuclei are stained blue. Magnification 600.

FIG. 3.—Transection of a blood vessel in the sub-cortical white matter—sleeping sickness. Only the neuroglial nuclei are stained. The lymphocytes are pale and unstained, and lie in the branching meshwork of the glia cells. Magnification 480. Eisath's stain.

FIG. 4.—Small vessel of brain of monkey in which the blood vessels of the brain had been rendered empty, and collapsed by ligation of all four arteries. This is to show the perivascular space filled with cerebro-spinal fluid, and the supporting neuroglial trabeculæ; such as are shown in the drawing are only seen at intervals. It can be understood that if these trabeculæ are greatly increased the lymphocytes will tend to be caught in the meshes. Magnification 500.

FIG. 5.—Shows macrophages (a) containing blood corpuscles, the result of a hæmorrhage into the cerebro-spinal cavity; lymphocytes (b), and diplococci (c), which are undergoing lysis. In the immediate neighbourhood could be seen crowds of diplococci and diplo-streptococci, which stained deep blue. Magnification 500.

FIG. 6.—Vessel of the brain with bacilli. Case 7, p. 30. Magnification 500.

PLATE IV.

FIG. 1.—Transection of cervical nerve close to the spinal ganglion, showing an infection of the sheath of the nerve by diplo-streptococci. The adjacent lymphatic glands showed points of suppuration. Magnification 200. (a) The micro-organisms, magnified 500. Case 69, L.L.

FIG. 2.—Vessel of the internal capsule of a case of acute sleeping sickness, with a large plug of cocci. Magnification 500. Stained by Gram's method.

FIG. 3.—Various degenerated cells seen in section of sterile lymphatic gland. Magnification 1,000. Leishman stain.

FIG. 4.—Lymphocytes and their transition to plasma cells *a*, *c*; *d*, degenerated plasma cell seen in section of lymphatic gland. Magnification 1,000. Leishman stain.

PLATE V.

FIG. 1.—Thread-like bodies and granules deeply stained, seen in section of lymphatic gland, probably altered and degenerated trypanosomes. Magnification 1,000.

FIG. 2.—Trypanosome in a lymphatic gland section amidst disintegrated cell products. Figs. 3 and 4 (Plate IV.), and figs. 1 and 2 (Plate V.), are drawings made from the same sections, 5 μ in thickness, stained with Leishman's stain and prepared from an enlarged cervical gland removed during life from a case (Bara Risgallah) of trypanosome fever, before symptoms of sleeping sickness had occurred. Magnification 1,000.

FIG. 3.—*Trypanosoma Gambiense* in smear of fresh gland juice, several lymphocytes, micronuclei. Magnification 1,000.

FIG. 4.—Section of lymphatic gland from a recently fatal case of sleeping sickness in a European. The glands in this case were not much enlarged. There is a very marked proliferation of the endothelial nuclei. Magnification 500.

FIG. 5.—Proliferation of the connective tissue cells of the reticulum of a lymph sinus; marked proliferation of the nuclei of the endothelial cells seen. This chronic change closely accords with the change observed in the perivascular lymph spaces of the central nervous system. Magnification 500.

FIG. 6.—Various granules and products of cell (and trypanosome?) degeneration seen in the perivascular infiltration of the central nervous system in sleeping sickness. Magnification 1,000.

PLATE VI.

Appearance of various pyramidal cells of the cerebral cortex in cases of very chronic sleeping sickness, showing various stages of chromatolysis and chronic degeneration. One cell is covered with phagocytes (*h*). Magnification 500.

PLATE VII.

FIG. 1.—Same section as that on Plate I., 4, more highly magnified, showing endothelial cell proliferation of the capsules of the posterior spinal ganglion cells and interstitial lymphocyte infiltration. Magnification 500.

FIG. 2.—Film preparation of Jinga trypanosoma in blood of infected monkey. Two trypanosomes are seen and three blood corpuscles. Beside there is a body, which appears as if fission were about to occur. Magnification 1,000.

FIG. 3.—Transection of a vessel of brain of ox that died of Jinga trypanosomiasis a short time after inoculation. A large number of chromatin rings are seen. Magnification 1,500.

FIG. 4.—Longitudinal section of a vessel of the same. Magnification 1500.

FIG. 5.—Bodies seen in a vessel of brain of ox. Some modified form of trypanosome? Magnification 1,000.

FIG. 6.—Splenic blood smear, showing Leishman Donovan bodies. Case of Kala-Azar somewhat similar appearance to 5. Magnification 1,000.

FIG. 7.—Spleen Kala-Azar, showing Leishman bodies in the form of definite chromatin rings. Note the similarity to the appearance presented by 3, 4 and 5. Magnification 1,000. Stained by Van Giesen's method.

PLATE VIII.

FIG. 1.—Longitudinal section of vessel of brain of ox that died of Jinga infection. Trypanosomes in various modified shapes are seen. Some of these may be amœboid forms of trypanosomes; probably some are trypanosomes which have been attacked by leucocytes. Magnification 500. Stained in bulk—methylene blue and eosine.

FIG. 2.—Small vessel of the medulla oblongata of rabbit inoculated with Surra. The animal died three months after infection. Shows a plasmodial mass in the centre and trypanosomes in a whorl near by. Magnification 1,000. Polychrome.

FIG. 3.—Nerve cells of above, showing chromatolysis, and a small vessel with the trypanosomes (*t*) coiled up, blocking it. Magnification 1,000. Polychrome.

FIG. 4.—Somewhat similar appearances as in fig. 2, seen in longitudinal section of vessel. Numbers of chromatin rings, probably macro-nuclei (A); (B) capillary blocked by trypanosomes; (C) trypanosomes in the tissue; (D) ganglion cell, showing marked chromolytic changes, probably due to capillary obstruction. The nucleus is swollen and clear, the body of the cell shrivelled, and there is an absence of Nissl granules. Magnification 1,000. Romanowsky.

PLATE IX.

FIG. 1.—Section of cortex showing pyramidal ganglion cells of Meynert's columns. It will be observed that the cells stain well, have retained fairly well a normal shape, and, considering the thinness of the section 5 μ, their numbers are not appreciably diminished. The lymphocyte and glia cell infiltration is not prominent in this region, although the specimen was made from the brain of a case of advanced sleeping sickness (Sempagama, Case 16, p. 33). Magnification 185.

FIG. 2.—Section of the cortex of a case of advanced sleeping sickness stained by Weigert method, to show condition of fibres. It will be observed that there is no gross fibre atrophy. Under a high power there is a diminution in some places, considerable of the tangential fibres and, to a less degree, of the super radial. Magnification 50.

FIG. 3.—Section of the spinal cord of Monkey 228. This animal died eight months after infection by fresh fly feeding. Observe the increase in number and size of the glia cells in the posterior column close to the posterior horn. There is also an accumulation of lymphocytes close to the ring of entry of the posterior root. These are seen somewhat indistinctly, owing to their being massed together. Magnification 170.

FIG. 4.—Section of spinal cord of very chronic sleeping sickness (Dreya, Case 6, p. 29). It shows no coarse tract degeneration, but under a higher magnification the most extensive subpial, septal and universal neuroglia proliferation can be seen. Magnification 7.

FIG. 5.—The neuroglial septal proliferation.

Plate X.

Fig. 1.—Central canal of 1st cervical segment of spinal cord, showing proliferation of ependymal cells to form glia cells. As the proliferation proceeds from within outwards, the ring of new young cells increases, leaving a more fibrillary substance behind in the centre, which fills up the canal. Around the ring of cells there is also a zone of a more fibrillary substance. The fibrils are the processes of the glia cells. Magnification 90.

Fig. 2.—Section of the heart of a case of advanced sleeping sickness which shows an accumulation of lymphocytes in the intermuscular lymph spaces. Magnification 250.

Fig. 3.—Section of the liver showing a chronic interstitial inflammatory change. There is accumulation of lymphocytes in the lymph channels of the portal canal. Magnification 180.

Fig. 4.—Anterior horn cell from a case of advanced sleeping sickness. The cell takes the basophile stain well, the Nissl granules are abundant in the body of the cell and on the dendrons. The cell infiltration around is mostly neuroglia, but there are lymphocytes. Magnification 540.

Plate XI.

Photographs of two Sleeping Sickness Patients (see Appendix, pp. 29-30).

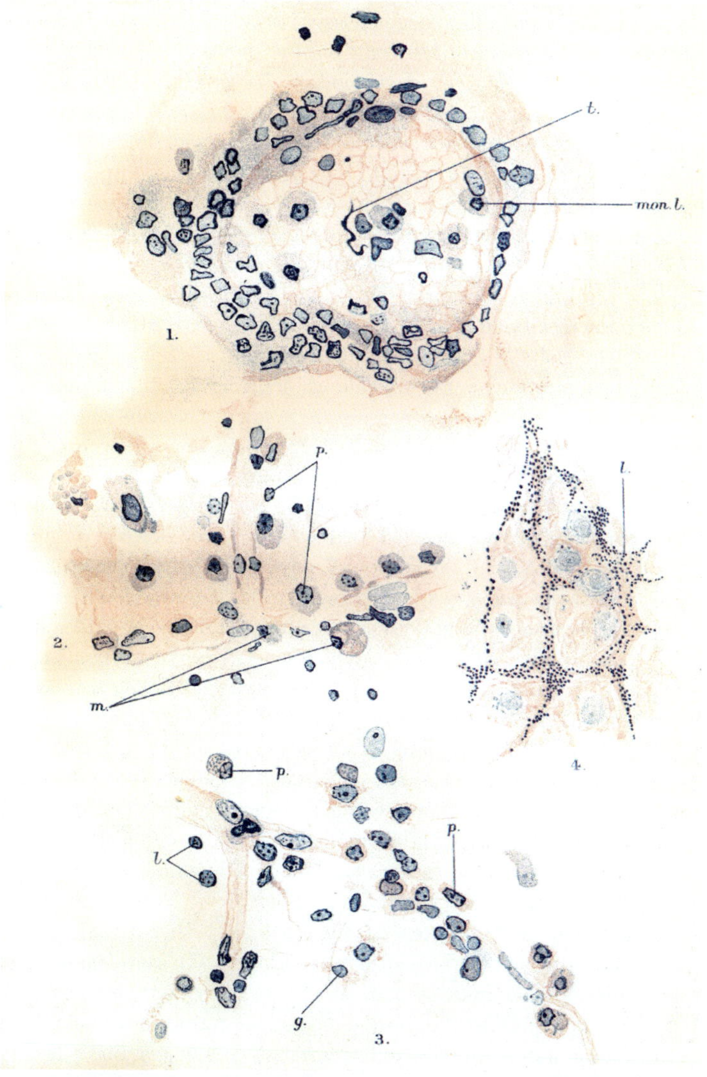

A. Kelley del.

Bale & Danielsson, L.td lith.

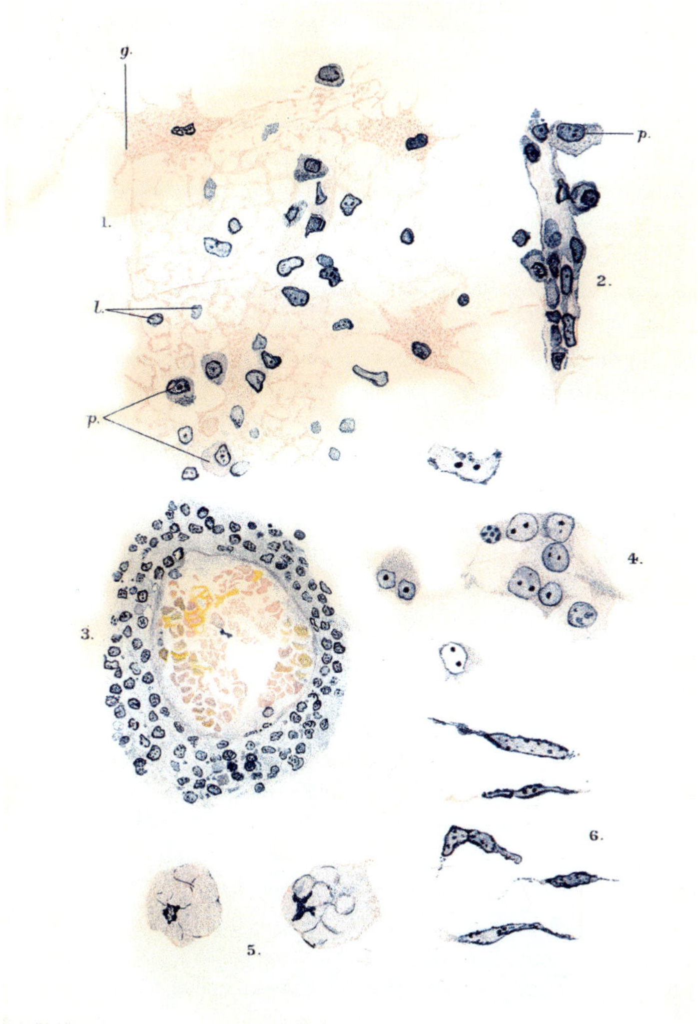

A. Kelley del.

Bale & Danielsson, L[td] lith.

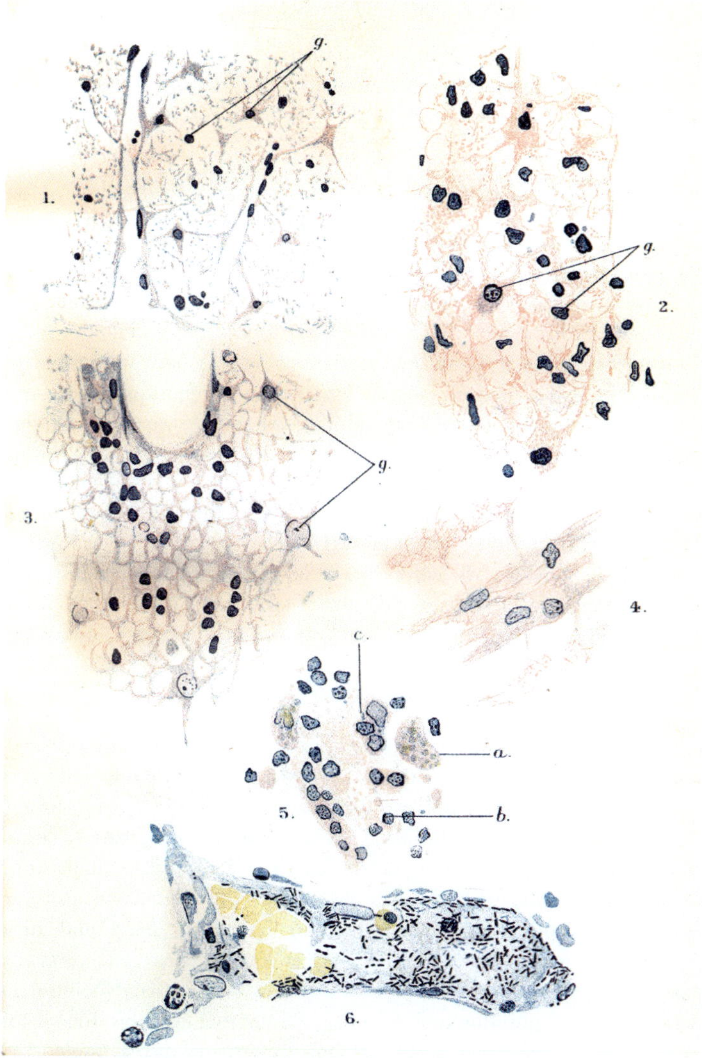

A. Kelley del. Bale & Danielsson, Ltd lith.

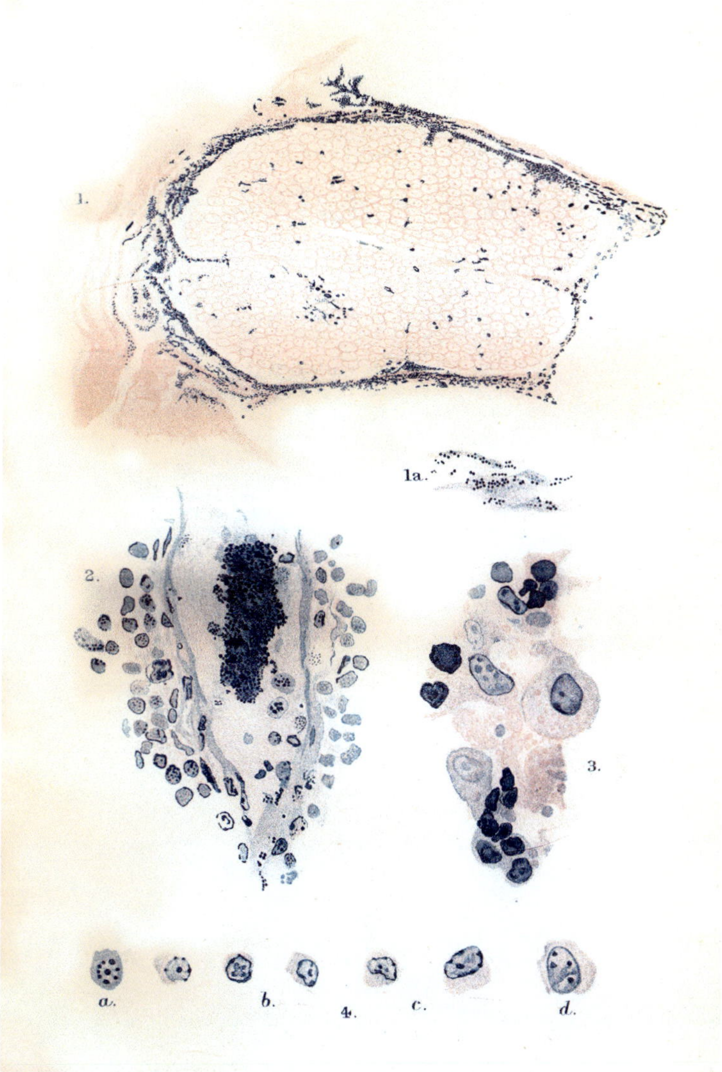

A. Kelley del. Bale & Danielsson. L^td lith.

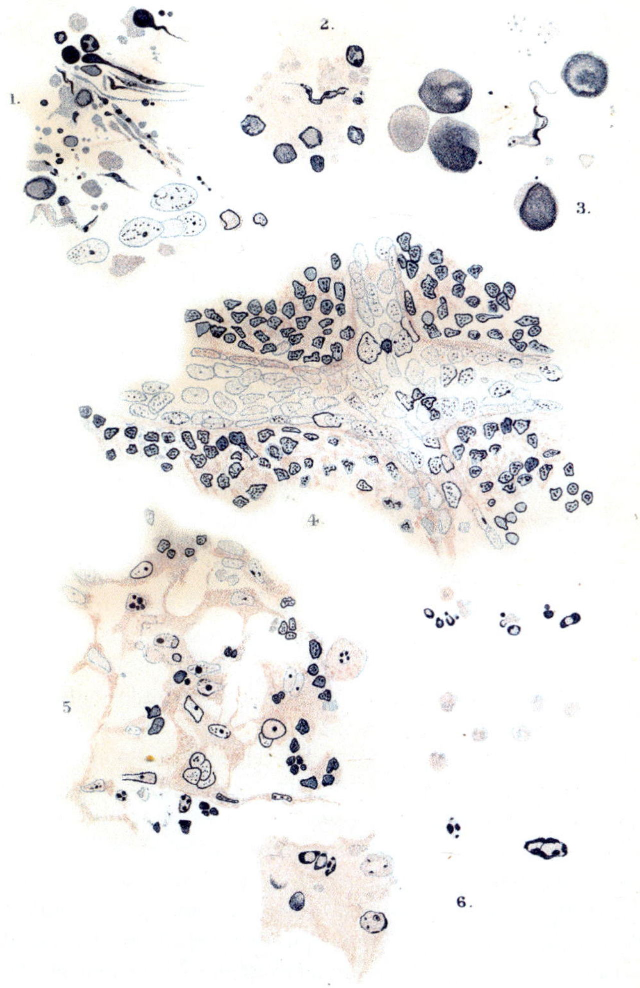

A. Kelley del. Bale & Danielsson, L[td] lith.

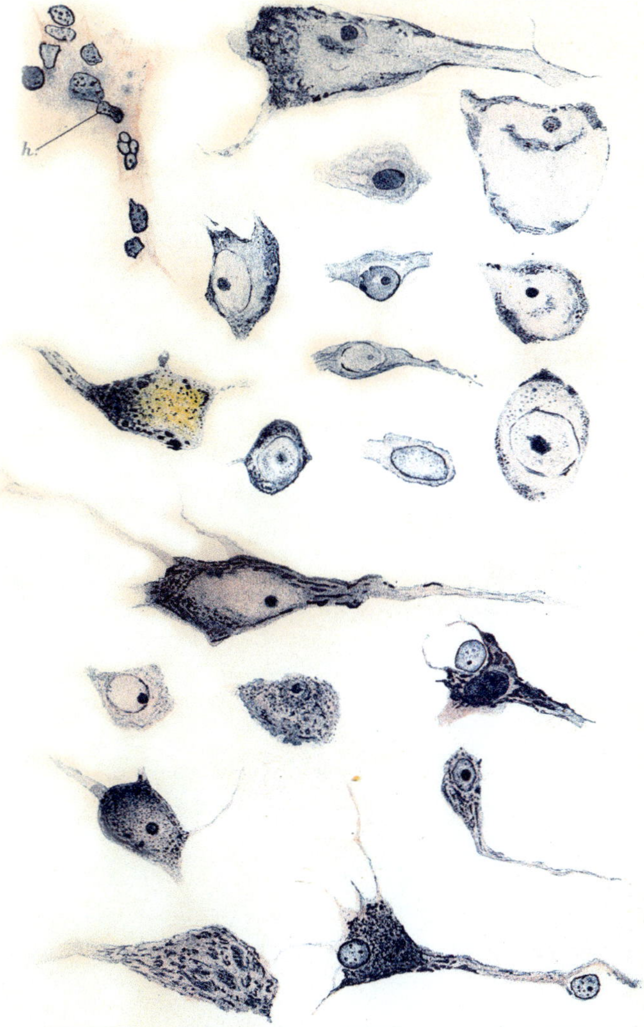

A. Kelley del. Bale & Danielsson, L^td^ lith.

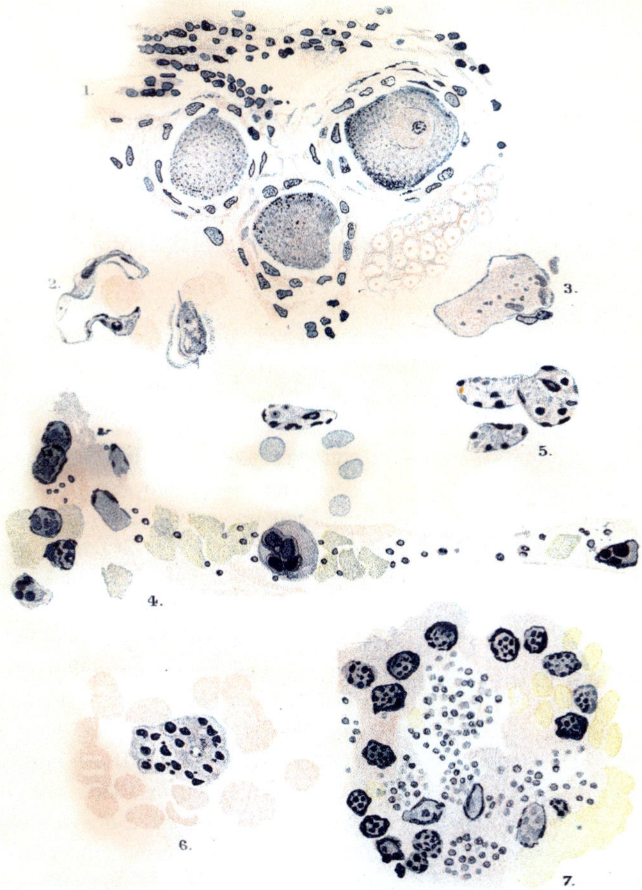

A. Kelley del. Bale & Danielsson, Ltd. lith.

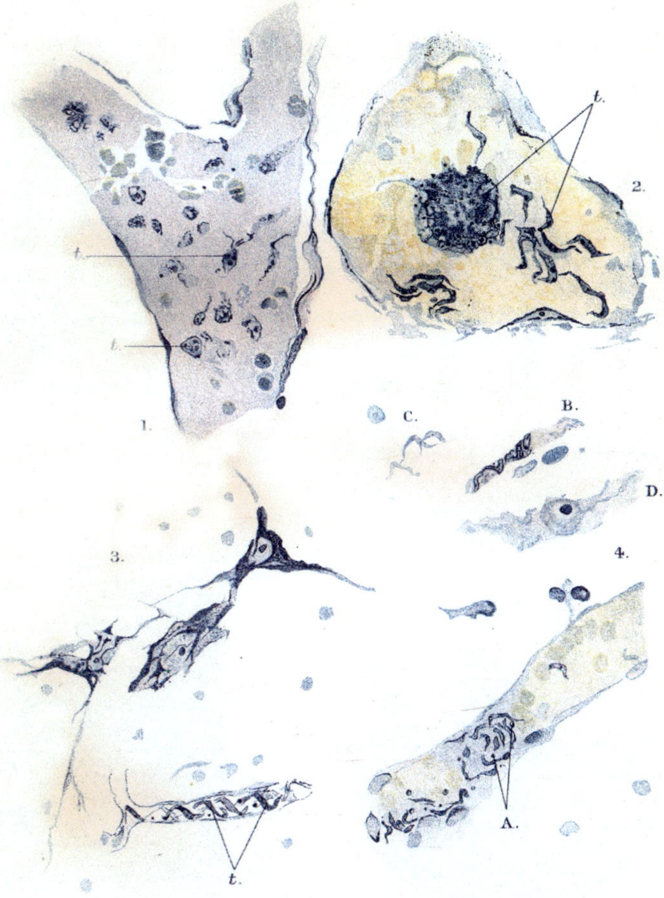

A. Kelley del. Bale & Danielsson, Ltd. lith.

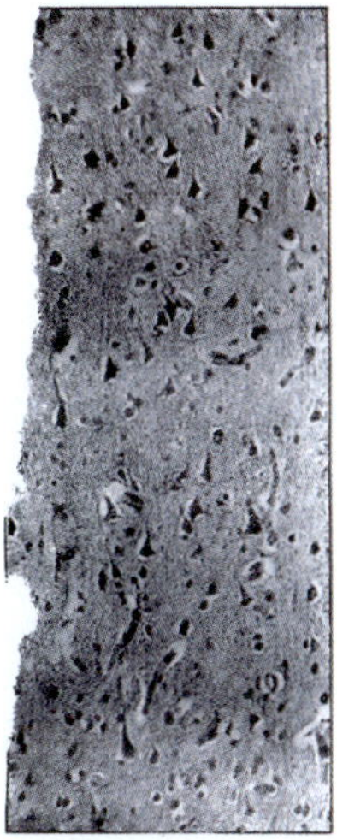

Fig. 1.

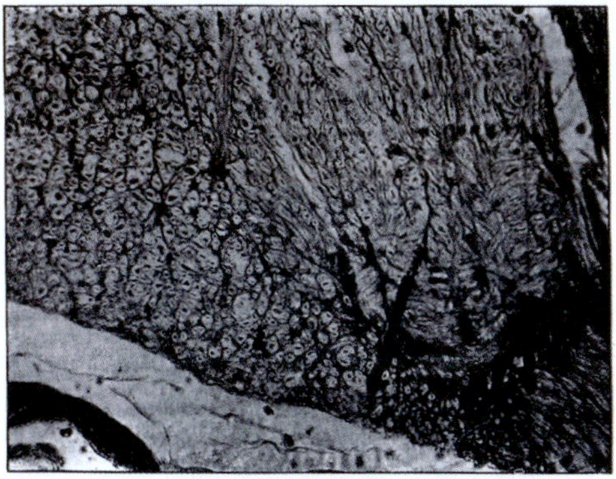

Fig. 3.

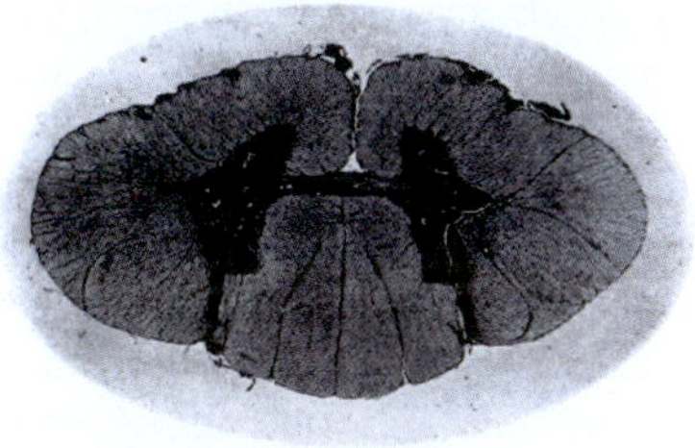

Fig. 4.

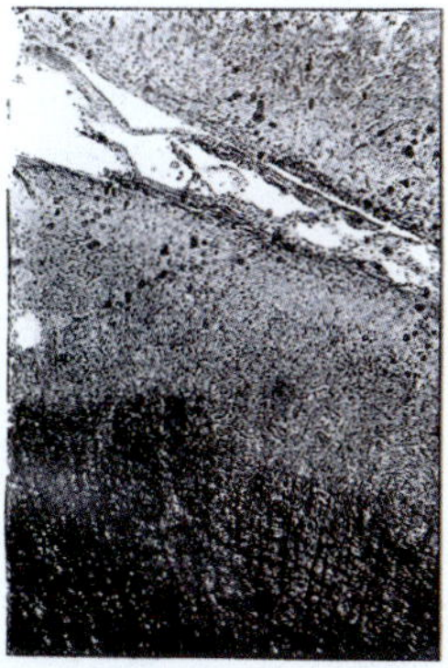

Fig. 2.

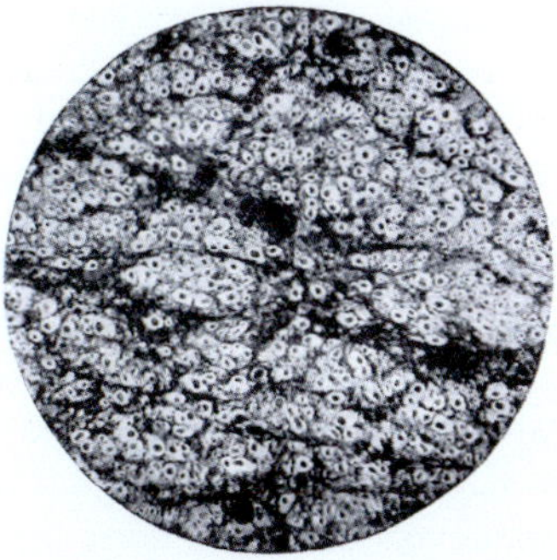

Fig. 5.

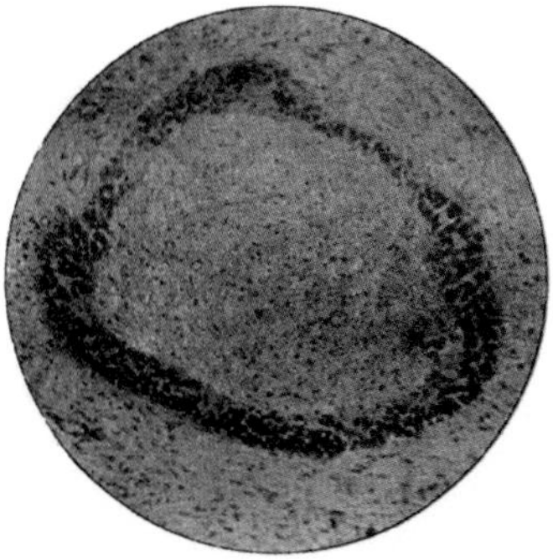

Fig. 1.

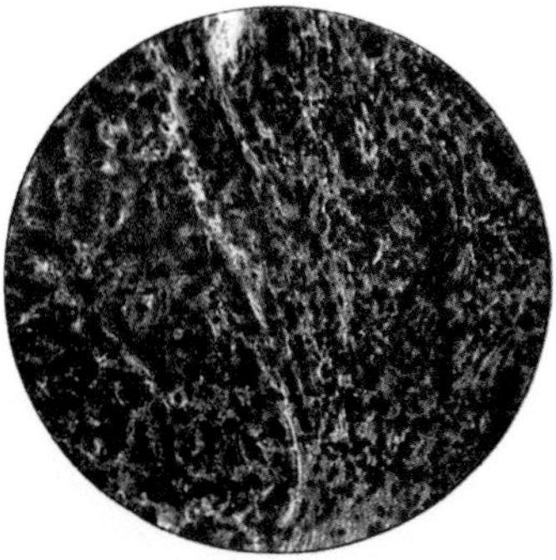

Fig. 3.

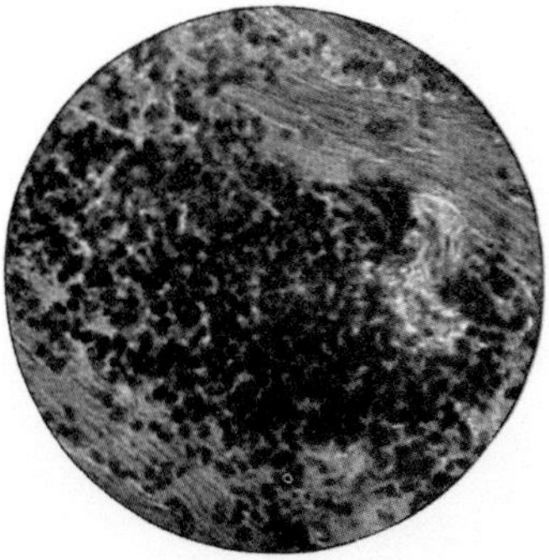

Fig. 2.

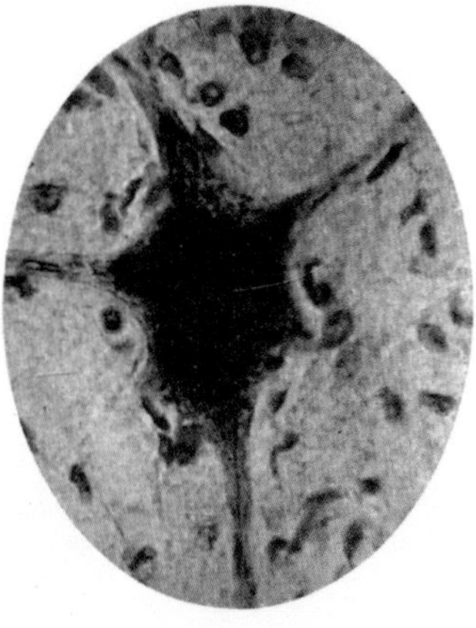

Fig. 4.

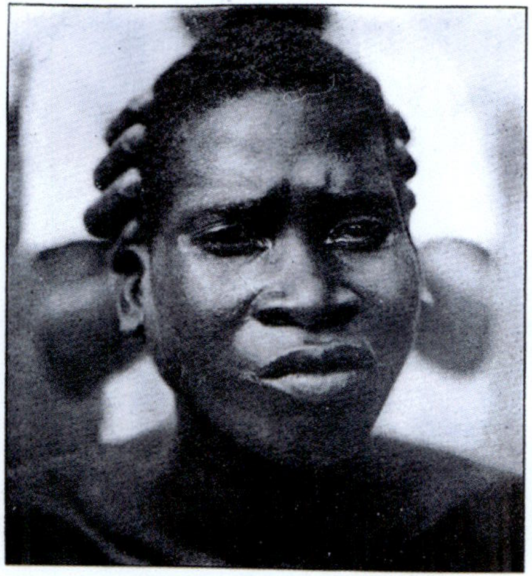

Fig. 1.

Photograph of an advanced case of Sleeping Sickness in a native, Mganda—"Dreya." An exposure of $\frac{1}{100}$ sec. with a "focal-plane" shutter was used, and even then it was found necessary to hold the head on account of the fine tremor present. Taken by Mr. R. J. Stordy.

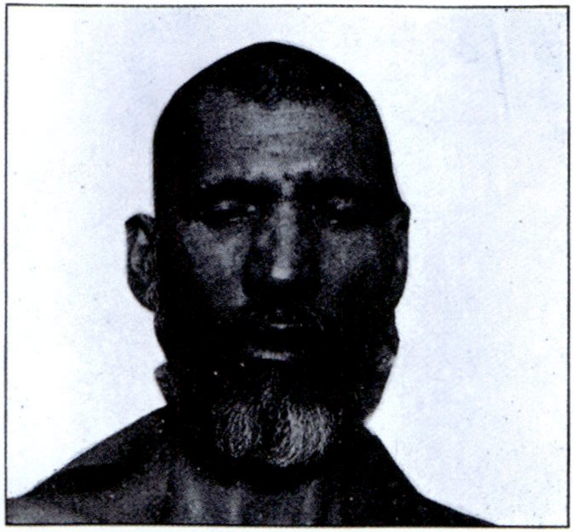

Fig. 2.

Photograph of a Persian suffering from Sleeping Sickness. Taken by Mr. R. J. Stordy, Government Veterinary Officer, Uganda and East Africa Protectorates. An exposure of $\frac{1}{100}$ sec. with a "focal-plane" shutter was used.

I am indebted to Dr. Nabarro for these two photographs, which exhibit in a striking manner the characteristic lethargic appearance which may be correlated with the advanced chronic interstitial meningeal and perivascular inflammation of the lymphatic system of the brain found in these two cases.

Printed in Dunstable, United Kingdom

91341565R00042